Best Trail Runs
San Francisco

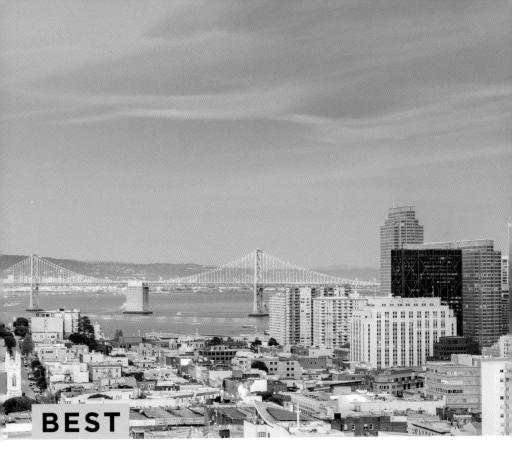

BEST
TRAIL RUNS
San Francisco

ADAM W. CHASE | NANCY HOBBS

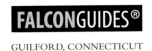

GUILFORD, CONNECTICUT

FALCONGUIDES®

An imprint of The Rowman & Littlefield Publishing Group, Inc.
4501 Forbes Blvd., Ste. 200
Lanham, MD 20706
www.rowman.com
Falcon and FalconGuides are registered trademarks and Make Adventure Your
Story is a trademark of The Rowman & Littlefield Publishing Group, Inc.

Distributed by NATIONAL BOOK NETWORK

Photo p. iii: iStockPhoto.com/vichie81; all other photos are by the authors.

Maps by The Rowman & Littlefield Publishing Group, Inc.

British Library Cataloguing in Publication Information available

Library of Congress Cataloging-in-Publication Data available

ISBN 978-1-4930-2522-0 (paperback)
ISBN 978-1-4930-2523-7 (e-book)

∞™ The paper used in this publication meets the minimum requirements of
American National Standard for Information Sciences—Permanence of Paper for
Printed Library Materials, ANSI/NISO Z39.48-1992.

Printed in the United States of America

Contents

INTRODUCTION

TRAIL RUNNING in the San Francisco area is about as diverse as its residents and cuisine. There are the rolling hills in the Marin Headlands offering iconic views of the Golden Gate Bridge, winding singletrack terrain in the North Bay, canopied forests and old-growth redwoods along the coastal areas, and countless wide-open spaces in the East Bay. The variety of terrain throughout the region appeals to a trail runner's discerning palate with gentle climbs to gnarly descents and everything in between. Runners here enjoy their trails year-round, some on misty mornings, others during a dry and sunny afternoon.

San Francisco's trails were the playground for the legendary Walt Stack, founder of the largest running club west of the Mississippi, the Dolphin South End Runners Club (DSE), who was one of the earliest "joggers' gurus" and known for the quote, "start slow ... and taper off." Stack ran so many marathons and ultras as well as all his regular training in the Bay Area from the 1960s through to the early '90s that he proclaimed, "I'm going to do this 'til I get planted." Having died in 1995, Stack's spirit is planted in the trails in this book and runs strong in the generations of runners he inspired.

We, too, are inspired by the Bay Area and its inviting off-road running that made it a true pleasure to conduct research for this guide. It was also a pleasure to work with our instrumental guides in the trail recon, with locals Richard Bolt, Robert Rhodes, and George Rehmet, who is also the featured runner on the cover.

We also provide guidance on gear, training, nutrition, and preparedness. *Best Trail Runs San Francisco* addresses running on wet ground and through water and mud, and the related concerns of exposure, traction, and other safety factors. The guide also discusses gear choices for addressing the various weather conditions you are likely to face on the trails we've included. Given our positions with the American Trail Running Association, we've also incorporated a discussion of when not to run on muddy trails, and environmental concerns that are unique to San Francisco trail running.

Difficulty Ratings

Being that many trail runners are also like Alpine skiers who understand the meaning of easy/green, intermediate (moderate)/blue, and difficult/ black for rating the difficulty of a run, we chose to go with that for the trails in this book. We acknowledge the subjective nature of this, noting that one person's hard is another's easy, but we did want to guide readers with some sense of relative ease or difficulty so that they may plan accordingly.

Cell Phone Coverage

We also deemed it helpful to readers to know if a trail has cell phone coverage. This is merely for safety purposes, and we caution that the signal is often carrier-dependent. We urge trail runners to use proper etiquette and to refrain from using phones, except in cases of emergency or to take pictures of the beautiful scenery through which these trails run.

Getting Started

Whereas road running is a more straightforward, linear function, trail running is multidimensional because it blends lateral motion with forward movement. To adapt your training routine to accommodate varying terrain inherent in trails, you will need to focus on strengthening your stabilizing muscles and balance. Similarly, because you will surely encounter hills—both steep and steady climbs—as a trail runner, you should consider the benefits of including training workouts that focus on strength, such as running hill repeats of varying intervals and distance. If you want to become a faster and fitter trail runner, you should consider increasing your speed through repeats, improving your fitness by running intervals and speed drills, and, finally, you may want to hit the weight room and incorporate a stretching regime.

Although one may experience relatively flat terrain in San Francisco, hills are more common, and Bay Area trail runners become quickly and painfully aware of the importance and benefits of hill training.

Pacing, or economy of effort, is probably the most important aspect of effective hill running. Much to their regret, novice trail runners are frequently less inclined (no pun intended) to use appropriate pacing on hills. As a result, they face the consequences of sputtering out with burning calves, huffing lungs, and possibly even nausea long before reaching the summit. Those new to hilly trails also tend to use improper form when descending and, accordingly, suffer from aching quadriceps and knee joints.

Running hills efficiently is a skill acquired through a process of fine-tuning and lots of practice, accounting for differences in body types, strength, weaknesses, agility, fitness, and aversion to risk. Armed with proper technique, a trail runner is prepared to take on hills—or mountains, for that matter—with alacrity instead of dread.

Whether you should attack with speed or power hike a hill or steep ascent is a complex decision that depends on the length of the climb, the trail surface, your level of fatigue, the altitude, the distance of the run, at what point in the run you encounter the hill, and whether you are training or racing. Efficient power hiking is often faster than running, especially in longer runs, when the footing is difficult, or at high altitude. It can be very rewarding to hike past someone who is trying to run up a hill and know that you are expending far less effort while you move at a faster pace. Conversely, it is quite demoralizing to be passed by a hiker while you struggle to run up a steep incline.

Two crucial elements of being a strong hill runner are tempo and confidence. Maintaining a smooth tempo on a hill requires focus as well as the ability to adjust stride length and cadence, also known as turnover.

Observing the fastest and most efficient climbers—both human and animal—it is easy to note their sustained turnover with a shortened stride on the climb. Even speedy mountain types go slower uphill and faster downhill, but the cadence of their legs hardly changes, regardless of the grade, the only difference being stride length. Just as you shift into lower gear when you bicycle up a hill, you need to shift gears as a runner by shortening your stride length.

Proper form and confidence on hills increases one's enjoyment of inclines and declines and, at the same time, decreases the chances of injury. With more confidence, you will be able to relax and run with a lighter, more flowing form that is more efficient and less painful. Knowing how to confront hills will keep you coming back for more, and because training on hills, whether on long, sustained ascents or shorter hill repeats, presents a superb opportunity for running-specific strength training, you will become a stronger and more confident runner overall.

TRAIL TRAINING

Compared with road running, trail running requires a more balanced and comprehensive approach, incorporating the whole body. Trail runners must be prepared to handle varying terrain, conditions, steep inclines and declines, and other challenges not found on the road. Fortunately, one thing trail runners don't need to train for is dealing with motorized vehicles.

Although many of the following training techniques apply to road running, it is also necessary to perform them on trails if your goal is to become a better, more accomplished trail runner. Yes, you may become a faster road runner by doing speed work on the track; but that speed does not always transfer to trails, where you will be forced to use a different stride, constantly adjust your tempo for frequent gear changes, and maintain control while altering your body position to stay upright.

DISTANCE TRAINING

If your goal is to run or race a certain distance, then training for that distance will be a mandatory building block in your trail training regimen. Incorporating long runs into weekly training will help your body adjust physiologically to the increased impact-loading stress by generating more bone calcium deposits and building more and stronger leg muscles and connective tissue. Building up weekly mileage improves your aerobic capacity to build up a base, upon which you can mix speed and strength training runs into your schedule.

Long training runs enable your body to cope with high mileage by breaking down fats for fuel and becoming more biomechanically efficient. Psychologically, long runs teach you to cope with fatigue. During lengthy training runs one experiences what can become an emotional roller coaster. It is useful to become familiar with how you respond under such circumstances, especially if you are training for a longer trail race. Long runs also help build confidence as a measure of progress and can become adventures into uncharted territory, allowing you to explore new stretches of trails and see new sights.

Some simple advice for those converting from roads to trails—especially for those who keep a log to record time, distance, and pace—is to forget about training distance or, if you know the distance of a trail, leave your watch behind when you go for a training run. Since trail running is invariably slower than road running, you will only get frustrated if you make the common mistake of comparing your trail pace with your road or track pace.

A prime reason for running trails is to escape tedious calculations, so free yourself from either distance or time constraints and just run and enjoy, particularly during your initial exposure to trail running. Tap into the wonderful feeling of breezing by brush and trees as you flow up and down hills and maneuver sharp corners with skill and agility. You can always fret about your pace as you develop your trail skills and speed.

If you base your trail-running training on the premise that long runs are primarily a function of time rather than ground covered, you should keep training runs close to the amount of time you think it will take to run your target distance. If, however, you are training for a trail marathon, you probably want to keep your distance training to less than the time it will take you to complete the race distance. To get there, you may want to set aside between one day every two weeks to two days a week for long runs, depending on your goal, experience, fitness background, and resistance to injury.

Trail runners usually dedicate one day of the week for a considerably longer training run, although some prefer to run two back-to-back relatively long days, especially on weekends when their schedules are more accommodating. This latter training method, known as a "brick workout," is common among ultramarathoners, who must condition their bodies to perform while tired and stressed. Newer runners should not try brick workouts until they are comfortable with trails and confident that their bodies will be able to withstand two days of long runs without breaking down or suffering an injury.

Because of the forgiving surface of trails, which may allow a person to run relatively injury free, newer trail runners are often lulled into building up their distance base with long runs too rapidly. Whether performed on road or trail, distance running takes its toll on the body; too quick an increase in distance often leads to injury, burnout, or leaving one's body prone to illness due to a compromised immune system. Depending on your age, experience with endurance athletics in general, and running history, it is better to increase your mileage or hours per week by no more than 5 to 10 percent per week.

Even if you increase your mileage base gradually, do not forfeit quality for quantity. Many runners succumb to the unhealthy game of comparing weekly mileage with either their previous weeks or those of other runners. Junk miles are just that. Depending on your objectives, it is usually better to run fewer miles with fresher legs and at a more intense pace than to slog through miles merely to rack them up in your logbook.

One way to check the quality of your miles is to wear a heart rate monitor and couple the distance of your runs with the goal of staying within your training zone at a steady pace. If you find your heart rate consistently rising above or falling below that target rate as you tack on the miles, that is a sign you are overtraining; and it is unlikely you will derive much benefit from those miles unless you are training for ultradistance.

SPEED TRAINING

For some trail runners, just being out on the trails and communing with nature is enough. They don't care about their pace. Building up one's distance base should help to increase running speed; but it only helps to a certain extent. To really pick up your pace and break through the barrier of your training pace, you should run fast. Running at a faster pace helps to improve both cardiovascular fitness and biomechanical efficiency. This discussion, however, is aimed at those who find it more exhilarating to push their limits, who enjoy the feeling of rushing along a wooded path, and who appreciate the fitness improvements that result from challenging themselves.

Beyond velocity, speed training—whether through intervals, repeats, tempo runs, fartleks, or other means—has positive physiological effects. Pushing the pace forces muscles and energy systems to adapt to the more strenuous effort of speed training. The body does this by improving the flow of blood to muscles, increasing the number of capillaries in muscle fiber, stimulating your muscles to increase their myoglobin and mitochondria content, and raising aerobic enzyme activity to allow muscles to produce more energy aerobically.

Running fast also provides a mental edge, because psychologically—if you are familiar with the stress and burning sensation known to many as "pain and suffering" that accompany running at a faster-than-normal pace during training—you will be able to draw from that experience and dig deeper into your reserves when needed during a race. Speed training on trails also forces you to push your comfort level with respect to the risk of falling or otherwise losing control on difficult terrain. Pushing the envelope helps establish a sense of confidence that is crucial to running difficult sections, especially descents, at speed.

Breaking away from the daily training pace and pushing oneself shakes up the routine and rejuvenates muscular, energy, and cardiovascular systems so that one may reprogram for a faster pace with more-rapid leg speed and foot turnover. Running at a quicker pace than normal helps to realign running form and teaches respect for different speeds.

However, because speed training is an advanced form of training, it should not be introduced into one's routine before establishing a consistent training base. Beginning trail runners should start by becoming comfortable with running on trails before they endeavor to run those trails fast.

Speed training stresses the body, so it may be wise to do your faster workouts on tamer trails with dependable footing, dirt roads, or even a track or road.

INTERVALS
Although interval training improves leg speed, its primary goal is cardiovascular—to optimize lactate threshold. As an anaerobic training tool, intervals are designed to increase one's ability to maintain a fast pace for a longer period of time. Without an improvement in lactate threshold, the runner will be unable to run or race a substantial distance at a faster pace than the rate at which the body can comfortably use oxygen, thereby causing lactate to form in the bloodstream. Intervals help to raise the level at which the body begins the lactate production process so that one is able to run faster and longer without feeling muscles burn or cramp. Upon developing a substantial training base of endurance, speed intervals allow acceleration of pace and an increase in overall running fitness.

Intervals are usually measured in terms of time rather than distance, especially if run on hilly or rugged trails. During the "on" or hard-effort segments of interval training, trail runners should work hard enough to go anaerobic (i.e., faster than one's lactate or anaerobic threshold so that the body goes into oxygen debt). During the "off" or recovery segments, you are allowed to repay some of the oxygen debt, but not all of it. The rest period should be sufficiently short so that you are "on" again before full recovery.

An interval workout may be a series of equal on-and-off intervals and recovery periods, or a mix of different-length intervals and recoveries. For example, a trail runner might run six intervals of 4 minutes, each interspersed with 3-minute recoveries. Alternatively, the interval session might mix it up with 5-, 4-, 3-, 2-, 3-, 4-, and 5-minute intervals, each separated by a 3-minute recovery.

Intervals may be as long as 6 minutes and as short as 30 seconds. Run intervals at a pace that is a bit faster than lactate threshold, which is usually equivalent to the pace run when racing a distance from 2 miles to 5 kilometers in length. The interval pace should be uncomfortable, but not excruciating; although not a sprint, you should feel you are running fast.

Run longer intervals if training for longer distances and shorter intervals if speed is the goal. The off, or recovery, period between intervals is an active rest that ranges between jogging and moderate running. Recovery time should be a little shorter than the time of the interval preceding it. In addition to recoveries between the intervals, any interval workout should integrate a substantial warm-up before and cooldown after running at or above lactate threshold pace.

HILL REPEATS AND REPETITION WORKOUTS

"Repeats" resemble intervals, except that leg speed and strength are emphasized more than lactate threshold (although repetition workouts have some beneficial lactate threshold effects). Put another way, repeat workouts are designed for biomechanical and physiological improvement more than for cardiovascular benefits. Hill repeats are intended to hone your climbing skills, and generally make for a stronger runner by taxing the muscular system with anaerobic intervals.

Repeats are run at or faster than lactate threshold pace, and each interval is shorter in length than a standard interval workout. Typically, repeats last 2 minutes or less; and because repeats are more intense than intervals, the recovery period is longer. Since the focus is muscle strength improvement rather than fitness, the active rest between repeats should be long enough to recharge and prepare for the next repeat at or above lactate threshold. In short, if you run a 2-minute repeat and need 3 minutes to recover, take the full 3 minutes. You want to recover enough to make each repeat interval sufficiently intense to realize the full benefits of the exercise.

Run each interval at a pace that you can maintain through the entire repeat workout. Don't push so hard during early repeats that you leave yourself unable to finish the rest of the workout. Hill repeats provide a great strength and lactate threshold workout with minimal stress to the body, because you push hard to go anaerobic while climbing but then rest as you slowly jog or walk to the bottom of the hill. Because of the reduced stress, you can throw hill repeats into your training schedule on a weekly basis without jeopardizing the health of your connective tissue.

TEMPO RUNS

Imagine a spectrum, with repeats that focus on biomechanics and muscular strength buildup at one end, intervals that focus on a combination of lactate threshold and biomechanics in the middle, and tempo runs at the other end, which emphasize lactate threshold or cardiovascular fitness.

Repeats   **Intervals**   **Tempo Runs**

├──┤

Biomechanics/Strength   **Cardio/Lactate Threshold**

Tempo runs are sustained efforts at an even pace, usually lasting about 20 to 40 minutes, although those training for longer distances may do tempo runs that stretch to 90 minutes. The pace should be a lactate threshold pace—which is faster than a pace at which one is able to maintain a conversation, but not faster than one that forces one to exceed 90 percent of maximum heart rate. The pace is one that could be maintained for about an hour, if racing. Since the goal of tempo training is to maintain a steady pace with consistent leg turnover, run tempos on a trail or dirt road that is relatively flat with good footing.

Tempo runs should include a warm-up and cooldown, both at a comfortable pace. If the tempo workout involves training partners, be careful to not turn the session into a race or time trial. To prevent that from occurring, wear a heart rate monitor and set it to sound an alarm if the heart rate rises above lactate threshold rate. Because tempo runs are physiological workouts, the goal is to run at a certain effort rather than to cover a certain distance. Depending on terrain, weather, and how rested you are beginning a tempo run, the pace may vary, but the body should nevertheless be working at threshold level throughout the workout.

Because considerable concentration and focus are required to maintain a steady lactate threshold pace for 20 minutes or longer, runners frequently find themselves a bit tired, both physically and mentally, the next day or two after a tempo workout. If that is the case, take a day of active rest or work a recovery run into your schedule. It may even be advisable to take the next day off to rest up and maintain trail-running vigor.

FARTLEKS

Fartlek is Swedish for "speed play." Scandinavians, known for their trail-running prowess and long history in the sport, pioneered the art of running fast on trails. Fartleks are creative workouts that weave a variety of paces into the same run. Although fartleks can be performed solo, they are often run as a group, in single file with the leader setting the pace—sometimes sprinting, sometimes jogging, sometimes walking, at other times simply running. Because the pace of a fartlek often varies with the terrain, these invigorating workouts are most successful if run on trails that offer a mix of short and long hills and plenty of turns and obstacles.

Fartleks offer a fun alternative to more standardized, timed speed workouts. Because they lack any regimented order, fartleks can reinject zip into a training routine that has grown boring, or introduce some excitement when running feels lethargic. The pacesetter can rotate, and faster runners may loop back to pick up stragglers to keep the fartlek group intact.

To capture some benefits of a fartlek when running alone, throw in some surges to get some speed training. Surges are short blasts of speed worked into a training run to accentuate a transition in the trail, such as near the top of a hill or when reaching the bottom of a hill and beginning a climb.

Another way to mix training with a little speed is to integrate striders or accelerations into the routine. An excellent time to insert some striders or accelerations is at the end of a trail run, just before the cooldown. Striders and accelerations are usually performed on flat, soft surfaces such as grassy parks, playing fields, or dirt roads. If striders or accelerations are run on grass or sand, try removing shoes so as to work on the muscle tone of lower legs and feet while feeling light and free in performing these speed workouts. Strider and acceleration distances should range between 50 and 100 meters, allowing for an additional 10 meters to get started and 20 to 30 meters to slow down.

A strider is usually run at a fast running pace, just under or even finishing with a sprint. Place emphasis on high knee lifts and getting a full kick off each step so as to cover as much ground as possible without overstriding. When striding, think of sprinters warming up on a track, swinging arms and lifting knees in an accentuated manner. Accelerations resemble striders, but begin more slowly and end in a full sprint.

"OFF-TRAIL" SPEED TRAINING

Although the goal of speed training is to improve physiology, the cardiovascular system, biomechanics, the muscular system, and mental strength, it is not necessary to do all speed training on trails. In fact, it is more effective to perform some speed training sessions on the track, dirt, or even paved roads. Depending on where you live and the types of trails to which you have access, it may be a lot easier to do speed training off the trails, reserving the trip to trails for longer runs.

Road and track are better suited for certain types of speed training. Tempo runs, where the focus is on a steady pace, and repeats, where the emphasis is on leg turnover, should be performed on flatter, more dependable surfaces. Roads or tracks are certainly easier than the trail for these types of workouts, especially if trails are icy or muddy.

Track sessions tend to be highly efficient. Perhaps it is the lane lines or bends of the turns, but there is something about running on a track that creates a feeling of running fast. That feeling may well convert to actual speed, which means a more effective speed session. Tracks are also useful because they are measured for convenient pacing. If one wants to do repeats or intervals and maintain a set pace, going to the track is an efficient alternative to the trail.

In addition to selecting the appropriate speed workout and venue to perform the session, also take the weather into consideration. If it is snowy, icy, muddy, or particularly windy, it may not be possible to get a good speed workout outside. Depending on training needs and personal preferences, train inside and run a set of repeats or intervals on the treadmill, or work on leg turnover with some spinning. However, many trail runners are adamantly opposed to such mechanical alternatives and insist on running outside, regardless of the weather. That is fine and well, but they then must be willing to either forgo speed training sessions when the weather is particularly nasty or attempt to do them under unfavorable conditions.

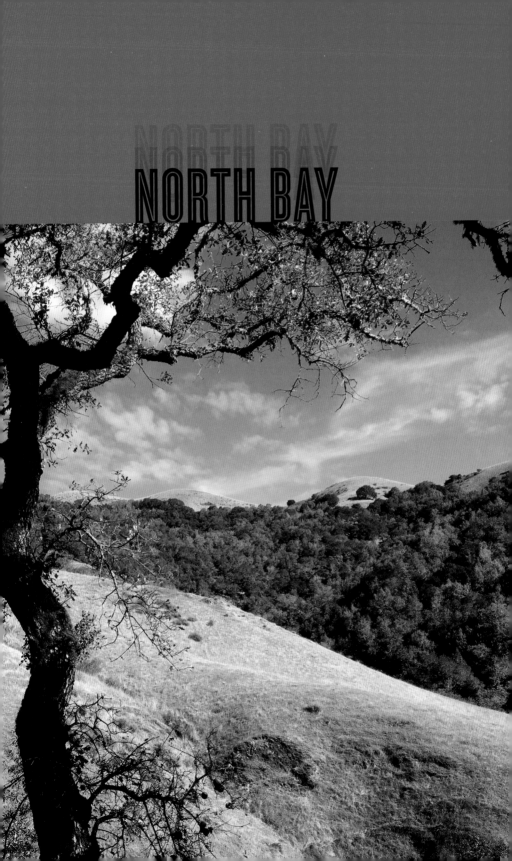

NORTH BAY

CHINA CAMP STATE PARK

LOCATED IN SAN RAFAEL, ON THE SHORE OF SAN PABLO BAY, China Camp State Park boasts more than 1,500 acres of terrain with 15 miles of trails. Although near an urban setting, this park is truly a hidden gem for trail runners, providing year-round training opportunities on singletrack and doubletrack trails complete with switchbacks, ascents, and descents.

6.9-MILE LOOP

THE RUNDOWN

START: Miwok Meadows Day Use Area; elevation 42 feet

OVERALL DISTANCE: 6.9 miles

APPROXIMATE RUNNING TIME: 80 minutes

DIFFICULTY: Blue. Easy, but boasts two significant climbs about 1.5 miles into the loop.

ELEVATION GAIN: 697 feet

BEST SEASON TO RUN: Because the trails have good runoff, year-round access

DOG FRIENDLY: Dogs are not allowed on the trails.

PARKING: Small fee, or purchase of an annual park pass, if you go through the tollbooth to park. Otherwise free on-street parking along North San Pedro Road (which requires a quarter-mile walk to the trailhead).

OTHER USERS: Equestrians, mountain bikers on most trails

CELL PHONE COVERAGE: Good

MORE INFORMATION: www.parks.ca.gov/?page_id=466

FINDING THE TRAILHEAD

From San Francisco follow US 101 north to North San Pedro Road in San Rafael (exit 454). Follow North San Pedro Road approximately 5 miles to the park entrance, which will be on the right side of the road. The

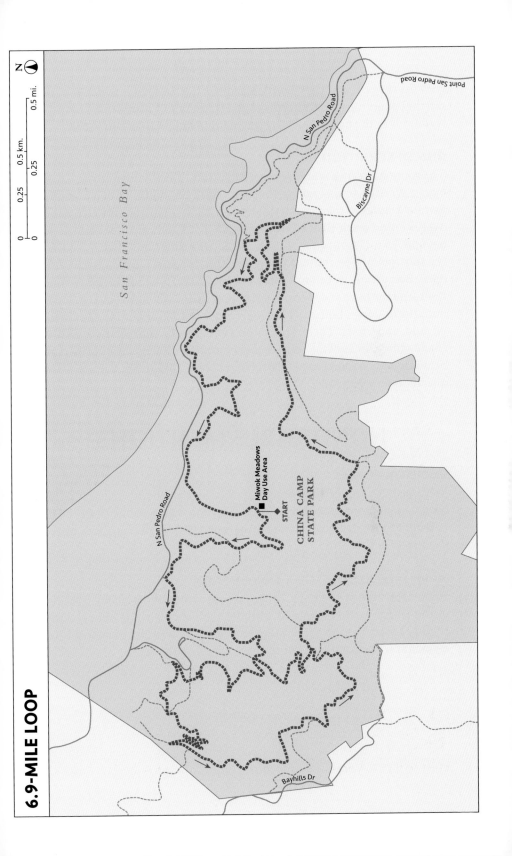

6.9-MILE LOOP

N

0   0.25   0.5 km.
0   0.25   0.5 mi.

San Francisco Bay

N San Pedro Road

Point San Pedro Road

Biscayne Dr

N San Pedro Road

Miwok Meadows
Day Use Area

START

CHINA CAMP
STATE PARK

Bayhills Dr

start for the trail is at the Miwok Meadows Day Use Area, which is a great starting point for numerous routes and is just one of many entry points to trailheads in the park, which is located just 4 miles east of San Rafael.

RUN DESCRIPTION

The route starts on a wide gravel roadway and quickly turns right to cross over a wooden bridge where the singletrack Shoreline Trail awaits. Follow for 2 miles to the intersection of Bay View Trail and stay left. At just over 3 miles, reach the Oak Ridge Drive Trail and continue east. At just beyond 4.5 miles, turn right back to the Shoreline Trail, looping back to the start point. The route is partly through forested terrain, partly in the open. Because of the canopy there is some cover in windy or rainy conditions, and the terrain underfoot is hard-packed—although rooted in spots— but affords good absorption during rainy months and limits the amount of mud underfoot. There are gentle switchbacks after a few quick yet challenging climbs. This route is a very rolling assortment of trails, some providing the opportunity to stretch out and quicken the pace. The final quarter mile is on road.

HONORABLE MENTIONS

5K OUT-AND-BACK

With just 266 feet of elevation gain, this gentle run on singletrack trails gives a quick intro to the park system. Start on the Shoreline Trail and run to Bank Ranch Fire Road for the turnaround back to the start. (See map on page 5.)

HALF-MARATHON TOUR OF THE PARK

With 1,850 feet of climbing, this route provides an excellent overview of the entire park system and includes the 6.9-mile route above, with a slightly longer loop on the western section of the trail and an out-and-back segment on the eastern side of the park. (See map on page 5.)

5K OUT-AND-BACK & HALF-MARATHON TOUR

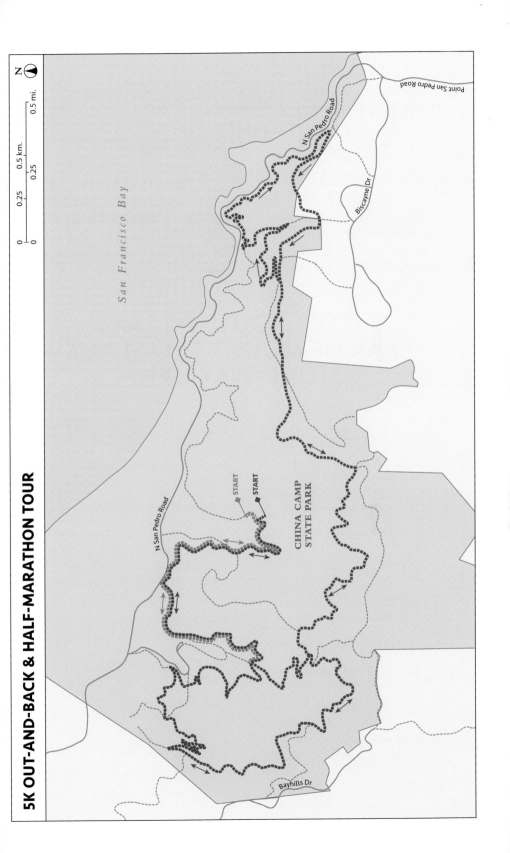

MOUNT TAMALPAIS

LOCATED IN THE HEART OF MARIN COUNTY, Mount Tamalpais (or "Mount Tam" to the locals) is a favorite of runners, hikers, and mountain bikers. Enjoy stunning 360-degree views of the Bay Area from the 2,571-foot peak. The West Peak of Mount Tam is 4 feet higher than East Peak, but there is no public access. From 1896 through 1929 steam trains carried passengers from Mill Valley to the Mount Tam summit.

DIRECT ROUTE TO EAST PEAK OF MOUNT TAMALPAIS (ONE-WAY UP)

THE RUNDOWN

START: The west side of the Marin County Fire Department building, Throckmorton Ridge Station; elevation 925 feet

OVERALL DISTANCE: 3.3 miles

APPROXIMATE RUNNING TIME: 45 minutes

DIFFICULTY: Moderate to strenuous

ELEVATION GAIN: 1,686 feet

BEST SEASON TO RUN: Year-round (except during storms/heavy rains due to the tall trees)

DOG FRIENDLY: No. The exception is service dogs. Dogs are allowed only on paved paths.

PARKING: Free. There is a parking lot opposite Mountain Home Inn. Another parking lot is just to the right of the fire station down the hill. But arrive very early on weekends and holidays to find space.

OTHER USERS: Mountain bikers, walkers

CELL PHONE COVERAGE: Excellent

TRAIL MARKINGS: Excellent

MORE INFORMATION: www.parks.ca.gov/?page_id=471

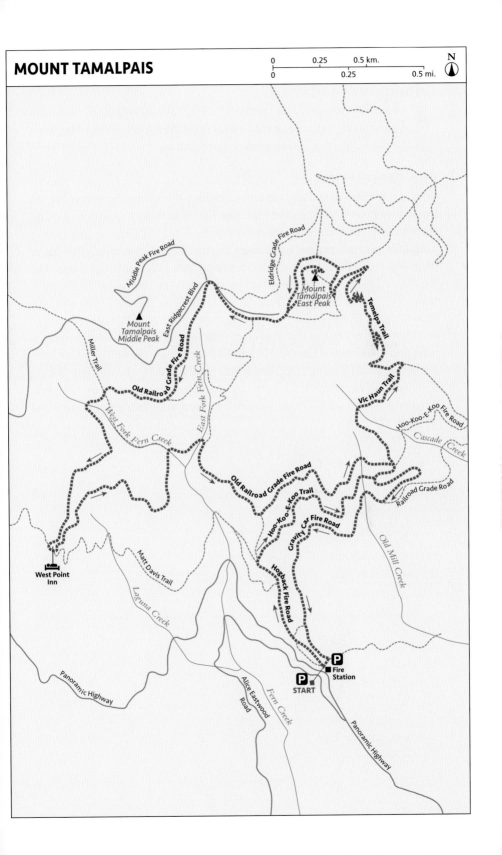

FINDING THE TRAILHEAD

From US 101 take CA 1 to Stinson Beach. Take a slight right turn onto Panoramic Highway. At 2.6 miles after Mountain Home Inn, turn right on Gravity Car Road toward the fire station.

RUN DESCRIPTION

Starting at the fire station, take the Hogback Fire Road, which is on the fire station's west side. Stay on the fire road for about a quarter mile and then turn right onto the Hoo-Koo-E-Koo Trail. At three-quarters of a mile, exit the trail and turn left to go on the Old Railroad Grade Fire Road for one-tenth of a mile. At the first intersection take a soft right onto the Vic Haun Trail, which is identified by its few steps. At the end of the trail, take a left up the Temelpa Trail. About 1 mile later the trail exits onto the paved Verna Dunshee Trail. Taking either a left or right will connect to the Plankwalk Trail as the trail circumnavigates the peak. Turning right provides views of the East and North Bays. Just past the Gravity Car Barn and water fountain, turn left up the Plankwalk Trail to the summit of 2,571 feet. Reverse the route for an out-and-back, or use the route on page 9 to descend on the Old Railroad Grade. Excellent trail markings ensure one stays on the route.

OLD RAILROAD GRADE (DESCENT)

THE RUNDOWN

START: Mount Tam summit; elevation 2,571 feet

OVERALL DISTANCE: 5.4 miles

APPROXIMATE RUNNING TIME: 50 minutes

DIFFICULTY: Easy

ELEVATION LOSS: 1,686 feet

BEST SEASON TO RUN: Year-round (except during storms/ heavy rains due to the tall trees)

DOG FRIENDLY: No. The exception is service dogs. Dogs are allowed only on paved paths.

PARKING: Free. There is a parking lot opposite Mountain Home Inn. Another parking lot is just to the right of the fire station down the hill. But you need to park very early on weekends and holidays to find space.

OTHER USERS: Mountain bikers, walkers, horses

CELL PHONE COVERAGE: Excellent

TRAIL MARKINGS: Excellent

MORE INFORMATION: www .parks.ca.gov/?page_id=471

(See map on page 7.)

FINDING THE TRAILHEAD

From US 101 take CA 1 to Stinson Beach. Take a slight right turn onto Panoramic Highway. At 2.6 miles after Mountain Home Inn, turn right on Gravity Car Road toward the fire station.

RUN DESCRIPTION

This particular run enables one to practice downhill technique. Because it requires starting at the summit, having someone drop you off at the top and pick you up at the bottom is advisable.

Starting at the summit, take the Plankwalk Trail down. At the bottom of the trail, take the paved East Ridgecrest Trail down. A quarter mile later, turn left onto the Old Railroad Grade Fire Road. Just at the 2-mile point, you will come to the West Point Inn. Turn left at the intersection to go around the other side of the inn and continue downhill on the same trail. At 4.3 miles stay to the right and go toward the Double Bow Knot by following signs to Mountain Home Inn. A tenth of a mile later, continue straight and enter the Gravity Car Fire Road. The trail will end at the parking lot below the fire station.

STRENGTH TRAINING

The image of a road runner is often that of the ectomorph—somewhat bony with elongated muscles and perhaps a sunken chest. Without besmirching those who restrict their running to paved surfaces, it can be said that trail runners tend to be a bit more muscular and "shapely" than their roadie equivalents. Many reasons account for the differences, but an important one concerns the trail runner's proclivity to vary exercise and recreation routines with other sports, many of which build strength and use one's upper body.

When not running, trail runners tend to gravitate toward other outdoor recreational activities, such as backpacking, rock climbing, swimming or pool running, mountain biking, kayaking, backcountry skiing, in-line skating, or even horseback riding. These other disciplines build strength and draw on muscles that are less or not often used when running. Many trail runners alter their workouts to combine trail running and at least one other outdoor activity. For example, a trail runner might run to the base of a mountain to do some bouldering. Another might mountain bike to reach a remote trail system, then quickly transition to running.

Trail runners can complement and enhance running strength with resistance training. Given that trail running draws from a broad range of muscles, the balance derived from regularly hitting the weight room as well as including a core strength program can have considerable performance-enhancing benefits, on and off the trail. Not only can one gain strength for speed and hill climbing through resistance training, but it serves to prevent injury, increase resting metabolism, align and balance muscles for improved biomechanics, and build tendon and ligament strength.

STINSON BEACH/ MOUNT TAMALPAIS STATE PARK/ GOLDEN GATE RECREATION AREA

STEEP RAVINE TO DIPSEA 10K LOOP

THE RUNDOWN

START: Parking lot near Stinson Beach; elevation 23 feet

OVERALL DISTANCE: 6.6 miles

APPROXIMATE RUNNING TIME: 80 minutes

DIFFICULTY: Blue

ELEVATION GAIN: 1,722 feet

BEST SEASON TO RUN: Year-round, but sections can be very muddy and slick in the rainy months.

DOG FRIENDLY: Yes

PARKING: Free

OTHER USERS: No horseback riders or bikes on this route

CELL PHONE COVERAGE: Good

MORE INFORMATION: www .nps.gov/muwo/upload/muir_ woods_pad_map.pdf

STEEP RAVINE TO DIPSEA 10K LOOP

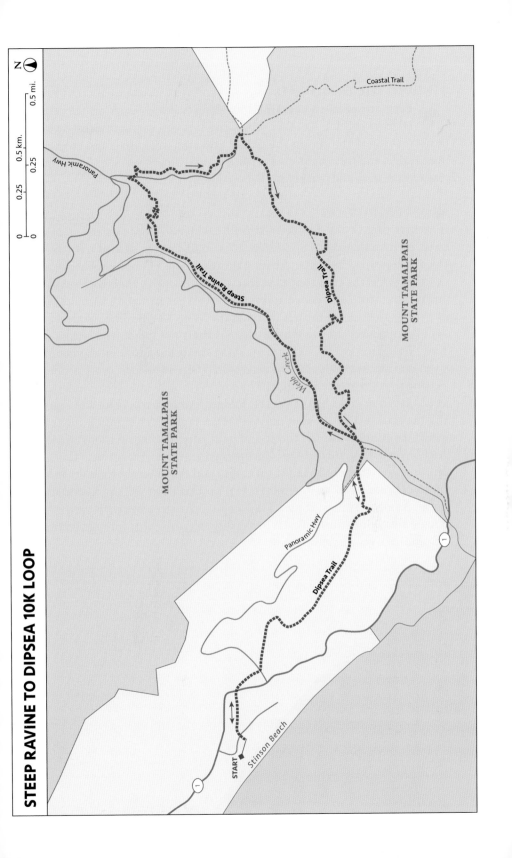

Coastal Trail

Panoramic Hwy

Steep Ravine Trail

Dipsea Trail

Webb Creek

MOUNT TAMALPAIS STATE PARK

MOUNT TAMALPAIS STATE PARK

Panoramic Hwy

Dipsea Trail

Stinson Beach

START

N

0   0.25   0.5 km.
0   0.25   0.5 mi.

FINDING THE TRAILHEAD

Park at one of the parking lots along Stinson Beach off Shoreline Highway/CA 1. Keep in mind, the lots get very crowded on the weekends. Start the run in the grassy area near the restrooms, cross the footbridge, and turn right on Arenal Avenue. Cross over Shoreline Highway to the trailhead marker for Dipsea Trail.

RUN DESCRIPTION

The first part of the doubletrack trail has many wooden steps to navigate, as the trail ascends up switchbacks, in and out of shaded trees, to an open meadow reached after crossing the road. After more switchbacks and wooden steps, the trail continues into the forest and again includes climbing on a mixture of wooden and rock steps. Approximately 1.4 miles into the route, the trail to the left becomes the Steep Ravine Trail, which you will follow. Keep an eye out for the possibility of fallen trees across the trail. There are several footbridges along the route and some tight turns over gnarled tree roots and exposed rocks. The bridge surfaces are prone to getting slick, so exercise caution. The route is mostly uphill for 3 miles and crests just after crossing the Pantoll Ranger Station parking lot and rejoining the trail, which becomes the Old Mine Trail. Turn right on the trail, which continues into the forest and gradually descends on long switchbacks over several footbridges. Once you emerge from the forest at Cardiac Hill at approximately 3.5 miles, turn right and then sharply right downhill on the Dipsea Trail for the return trip on this keyhole loop to the start point. Along the famed Dipsea Trail, enjoy open stretches with views—on a fogless day—of Stinson Beach in the distance, as well as forested sections descending over numerous steps.

MOUNT TAM WATERSHED

OWNED BY THE MARIN MUNICIPAL WATER DISTRICT since its acquisition in 1912, the Mount Tam Watershed covers nearly 19,000 acres and is adjacent to other open space and recreational lands, including the Golden Gate National Recreation Area, Point Reyes National Seashore, Muir Woods National Monument, Samuel P. Taylor State Park, Mount Tamalpais State Park, Marin County Open Space lands, and other local and county park lands. There are several entry points to the park from Fairfax, Ross, and Mill Valley to enjoy more than 57 miles of trails and fire roads. Within the trail system, 17.8 miles are designated for equestrian use. Fire roads are mountain bike friendly. The trails are very well signed.

4.1-MILE KEYHOLE LOOP

THE RUNDOWN

START: Parking lot at end of Lagunitis Road; elevation 94 feet

OVERALL DISTANCE: 4.1 miles

APPROXIMATE RUNNING TIME: 50 minutes

DIFFICULTY: Green

ELEVATION GAIN: 548 feet

BEST SEASON TO RUN: Year-round. Avoid in heavy rains.

DOG FRIENDLY: Leashed dogs

PARKING: Free, but limited spaces near this trailhead. On weekends waiting 15 minutes or more for a parking space is not uncommon.

OTHER USERS: Mountain bikers and equestrians

CELL PHONE COVERAGE: Good

MORE INFORMATION: www .marinwater.org/137/ Watershed

4.1-MILE KEYHOLE LOOP

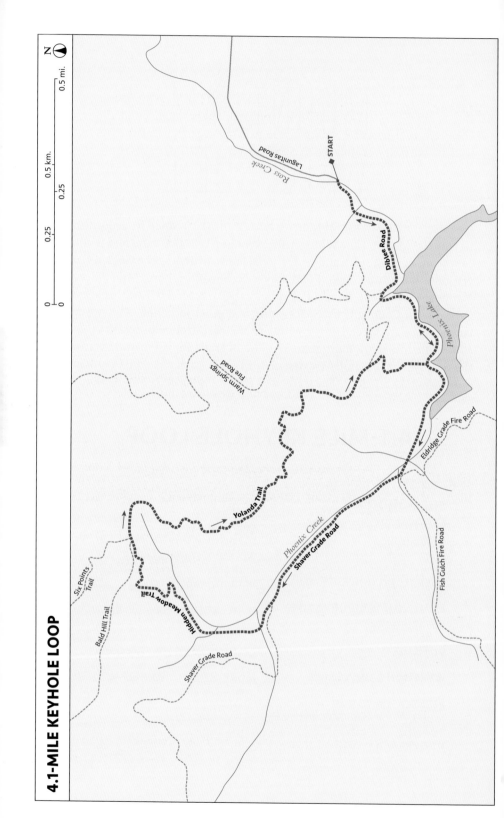

START

Lagunitas Road

Ross Creek

Diblee Road

Phoenix Lake

Warm Springs Fire Road

Yolanda Trail

Eldridge Grade Fire Road

Phoenix Creek

Shaver Grade Road

Fish Gulch Fire Road

Six Points Trail

Bald Hill Trail

Hidden Meadow Trail

Shaver Grade Road

N

0   0.25   0.5 km.

0   0.25   0.5 mi.

FINDING THE TRAILHEAD

From US 101 head west on Sir Francis Drake Boulevard in Greenbrae. Turn left on Lagunitas Road and park at the small lot at the end. There are two portable toilets in the parking area. Start at the wooden bridge by the interpretive signage and turn left up the fire road.

RUN DESCRIPTION

Follow the fire road (Shaver Grade Road), keeping Phoenix Lake (one of the five human-made reservoirs in this watershed) on your left. About three-quarters of a mile past the lake, turn right on singletrack trail at the signpost for Hidden Meadow Trail. The trail briefly runs parallel to the fire road before meandering to the right over a footbridge and then up a few tight switchbacks in the forest before reaching an open area. After the forest, the views that await after the short climb are fantastic. Glimpses of Mount Tam in the distance and rolling hillsides delight the senses in this very serene and peaceful setting. Continue on the Hidden Meadow Trail to the junction of the Yolanda Trail, approximately 2 miles into the run. Take the left junction for a longer route toward Bald Hill, or the junction to the right back to the fire road on a rolling but mostly downhill singletrack. At

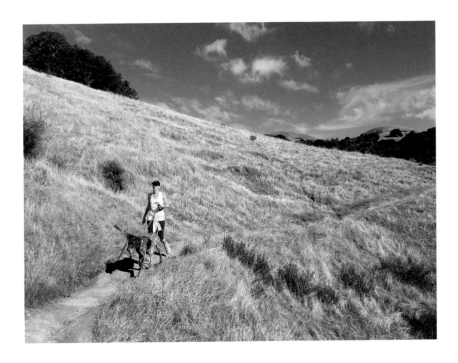

the fire road (Shaver Grade Road), turn left and head back to the parking lot for this 4.1-mile keyhole loop. If you have the time and energy, explore other trails in this area as they lead and connect to more open space opportunities to the north and west.

STRETCHING

Although athletes have focused on flexibility for decades, coaches and trainers have only recently begun stressing the importance of stretching (though some discourage the practice).

Stretching used to be something smiling people wearing leotards did in black-and-white television programs while they bounced in what has become an antiquated school of ballistic stretching: "And one ... two ... three ..." Since those days, the art of stretching has grown dramatically, and trail runners may now choose among myriad techniques.

Stretching is fundamental to gaining and sustaining flexibility, which is a crucial element of trail running. By maintaining a regular stretching routine, trail runners are able to help their muscles, tendons, and ligaments remain supple to avoid injury. Stretching staves off stiffness and rigidity brought on by training and racing, and increases elasticity and resilience of connective tissues. Stretching also aids in recovery, injury prevention, stride length, strength, and nimbleness on the trail.

There is a great diversity in stretching philosophies, and each school of thought has its own set of guidelines. The following recommendations for the trail runner were gleaned from an examination of these various approaches to stretching:

- Warm up before stretching. Warm muscles are less prone to strains, pulls, rips, or other injuries. Depending on the temperature outside, the location of the warm-up, the particular warm-up exercise, and its intensity, the pre-stretch period should be approximately the time that you would take to cover a flat mile. And do some stretching after the run to prevent post-workout soreness.

- Use proper form to isolate particular target muscles. If questions arise about how to go about a specific stretching routine, take a stretching class at a local health club or recreation center, consult with a personal trainer or coach, or check a book on stretching. Bob Anderson's 1975 book *Stretching* remains one of the better texts on the subject. Build a repertoire of stretches that addresses your particular needs, and stick to it as a regular part of your training schedule.

- Don't bounce. Ballistic stretching triggers a reflex that has the effect of tightening muscles. Ballistic stretching may also lead to a strain or other damage caused by bouncing beyond the natural range of motion. Using a long, sustained static stretch after warming up releases tension that has built up in the area of focus.

- Isolate particular muscles that are the goal of a particular stretch, and "breathe" into specific muscles as you feel slow elongations of the targeted area. Stay relaxed and use slow, rhythmic breathing. Hands, feet, shoulders, jaw, and face should not reflect tension.

- Continue the stretch to the point where a slight pull is felt, but not to the point of pain. According to Anderson, a mild comfortable stretch should result in tension that can be felt without pain. Do not gauge a stretch by how far you can reach; go by feel alone.

- If you are susceptible to particular types of injury or are currently injured, pay special attention to stretching that area. In some cases, stretching may make the injury worse or prolong recovery. It may be worth consulting an expert before engaging in any stretching routine while injured.

- When performing a static pose, hold the stretch for as long as 30 seconds and stretch both sides equally. Anderson recommends that when doing a stretch, you should feel comfortable enough with the tension that can it be held for 10 to 25 seconds, after which the initial feeling of the stretch should subside or disappear. That kind of stretching reduces muscle tension and maintains flexibility.

- To increase flexibility, Anderson recommends a "developmental stretch." After an easy stretch to the point where the feeling of tension dissipates, go into the pose again—but go deeper—until increased tension is felt. The stretch should not feel any more intense when held for 10 to 30 seconds. If it does, ease off to a more comfortable position.

- Incorporate the above rules as you customize a stretching routine that fits and appeals to your particular needs.

Consider incorporating some of the following stretches into your stretching regimen as a trail runner. These suggestions are by no means exhaustive, and it is recommended that additional resources be consulted to select and perfect an appropriate personal stretching routine.

Hamstrings: A modified hurdler's stretch involves sitting with one leg bent and that foot tucked against the inside of the thigh of the extended leg. From that position, lean forward (keeping the back straight) from the hips to touch with one or both hands the foot of the extended leg, reaching until tension is felt in the hamstring of the extended leg. Another hamstring stretch is to lie flat on your back, lift one leg, and pull it toward the chest, with the other leg bent and its foot planted straight in front. A third hamstring stretch is to stand with one leg raised so that foot rests on a solid object, such as a stool or a rock that is about at knee level. With the standing leg slightly bent, lean forward from the hips, keeping the back straight, and reach for the ankle of the extended leg until stretch is felt in the hamstring of the extended leg.

Iliotibial (IT) Band: The band that stretches from just behind the hip, running down the side of the leg and connecting to the top of the shin, is the IT band. When the IT band tightens, it can cause a flare-up on the side of the knee, resulting in pain. If a runner persists in running with a problematic IT band, it can ultimately seize up like an engine that has run dry of lubrication.

Any one or all of the following stretches can keep the IT band loose and flexible. In a sitting position with both legs stretched in front, cross one leg over the other and cradle the crossed leg in your arms, pulling the shin and foot of the crossed leg toward the chest until stretch is felt in the hip of the bent leg. For a deeper stretch, cross the other leg over the extended leg, placing the foot of the bent leg on the other side of the extended leg and placing the opposite elbow against the bent knee (e.g., if the left leg is bent, place the right elbow against the left side of the left knee), and press against the bent knee until the stretch is felt. Or, from a standing position, cross one leg in front of the other and lean forward to touch the toes until tension is felt in the hip of the rear leg. In the same pose, stand more upright and lean into the hip of the rear leg until tension is felt.

Groin: Because trail runners consistently have to dodge obstacles on the trail, they must incorporate considerably more lateral motion than do road runners. Sudden movement from side to side can lead to strain in the groin unless that area is properly limber. One easy stretch is to sit down, pull both heels into the groin, and place the soles both feet against each other, with knees close to or touching the ground. Increase the tension of the stretch by pulling the heels closer to the body or lowering the knees to the ground by pressing elbows against knees.

Quadriceps: Descending a rocky trail at a fast pace places considerable stress on the quadriceps. A number of stretches can be performed to loosen your quads. One easy stretch is to stand on one foot and bend the other leg backward, reaching back with both hands to hold the foot of the bent leg, lifting the foot to the point where a stretch is felt. Another stretch is one that should not be performed by those with week ankles or problem knees—if in doubt, consult an expert. Kneel on the ground with both knees, feet pointed backward and tucked underneath. Lean backward until the quads feel a stretch. Another basic quad exercise that helps to build flexibility is to perform a static squat by slowly bending the knees while keeping the back straight and your weight centered over your pelvis.

Calves: Non-runners often chuckle at the sight of runners who appear to be trying to push over a building or lamppost. Little does the non-runner know that the runner is merely stretching calf muscles. This stretch involves standing about an arm's length from a wall, post, tree, rock, or other fixed object and placing both hands against the object. Bend one leg off the ground as the other leg is stretched straight behind, keeping the heel of the straightened leg on the ground with the toes facing forward. Lean into the rear leg until that calf is stretched.

Devoting substantial time to stretching calves may be well worth the investment, especially if focus is on the full range of the gastrocnemius muscles. Maintaining calf flexibility is very important for trail runners who tend to run high on their toes or do a lot of hill work. For those limber enough to touch their toes, another way to stretch the calves is to sit on the ground and extend both legs parallel straight in front. Lean forward from the hips with back straight and hold the toes, pulling them toward the body until a stretch is felt in the calves. If you cannot touch your toes, loop a band or towel around your toes, then pull on it to stretch the calves.

Ankles and Achilles Tendons: One of the greatest problem areas for trail runners is weak ankles. Maintaining flexible ankles helps prevent ankle rolls or sprains and enables you to recover from what could be a calamity. Ankle rotations are easy to perform and can be done even while sitting. Lift one foot a few inches off the ground and slowly rotate it through its full range of motion. Rotate in both directions. To stretch the Achilles tendon, stand with one leg raised so that its heel rests on a solid object that is about at knee level. Lean forward, place both hands under the ball of your raised foot, and gradually pull toward the body. After feeling the stretch, point the toes toward the ground as far as possible.

Back and Trunk: Trail runners should invest heavily in a limber back and trunk. A tight back or midsection can lead to a nightmare of injuries, terrible running form, and an unhealthy posture. Practicing yoga on a regular basis can lead to a flexible back and relaxed running form. Back and trunk stretches include a standing waist twist, where hips are rotated in one direction as you look over your shoulder and hold the stretch, with hands on hips, knees slightly bent, and feet pointed forward. For a standing back extension stretch from the same standing position, place the palms just above the hips with fingers pointing down, then slowly push the palms forward to create an extension in the lower back, and hold the stretch.

Another easy back stretch that releases tension that may build up from running hills or rocky trails is to lie on your back and bend your knees, lifting them slowly toward your chest until you can clasp your hands around your shins. Keep pulling the knees into the chest until the lower back feels stretched. An additional lower back stretch involves lying on your back with one leg extended flat on the ground. Bend the knee of the other leg and cross it over the extended leg, using the arm on the side of the extended leg to gently pull the bent knee down toward the ground, keeping both shoulders flat until a stretch is felt.

Upper Body: Because trail runners tend to use their arms more than road runners, due to the need for balance and occasional trail touchdowns or scrambling, it is more important to keep your arms loose. The same goes for a trail runner's neck and shoulders. Long ascents or descents can cause trail runners to tense up the upper body. The advantage of most upper body stretches is that they can be done on the fly, providing relief without the need to stop. If you grow tense during a run, try flapping your arms about wildly, throw your head to and fro, and jut your hips around in a very silly display. In addition to laughing at yourself—and encouraging anyone in sight to laugh as well—this odd behavior releases built-up stress and at least temporarily realigns running form into a more relaxed and efficient posture.

To loosen tight shoulders and lower neck tension, incorporate slow-moving "windmills" (shoulder rotations with swinging arms) and exaggerated yawning-type movements in both directions. Rotate your head around in all directions, but be careful in trying this on a run, since it tends to momentarily compromise balance. For a more intense stretch, apply pressure on your head with your hands as the head is rotated. For good measure, throw in some shoulder shrugs, lifting the shoulders up toward the ears. To loosen arms and shoulders, raise one at a time, folding it at the elbow behind the head while using the other arm to gently apply pressure so that the hand of the bent arm flows down the upper back.

POINT REYES
NATIONAL SEASHORE

LOCATED IN MARIN COUNTY, the Point Reyes National Seashore boasts more than 71,000 acres, many of which are on the 80 miles of shoreline. The area has about 150 miles of trails, with a high point realized at Mount Wittenberg, measuring 1,407 feet. Stay on the trails to avoid encounters with poison oak, stinging nettles, ticks, and yellow jackets.

THE RUNDOWN

START: Bear Valley Visitor Center; elevation 117 feet

OVERALL DISTANCE: 5.3 miles

APPROXIMATE RUNNING TIME: 70 minutes

DIFFICULTY: Blue

ELEVATION GAIN: 1,290 feet

BEST SEASON TO RUN: Year-round

DOG FRIENDLY: No

PARKING: Free

OTHER USERS: Equestrians on designated trails

CELL PHONE COVERAGE: Good

MORE INFORMATION: www .nps.gov/pore/planyourvisit/ beaches.htm

FINDING THE TRAILHEAD

There are several parking areas at the Bear Valley Visitor Center on Bear Valley Road, located just northwest of CA 1 in Olema. There is also public transportation to this location. The trailhead is located at the far west end of the parking lot, identified by a gate.

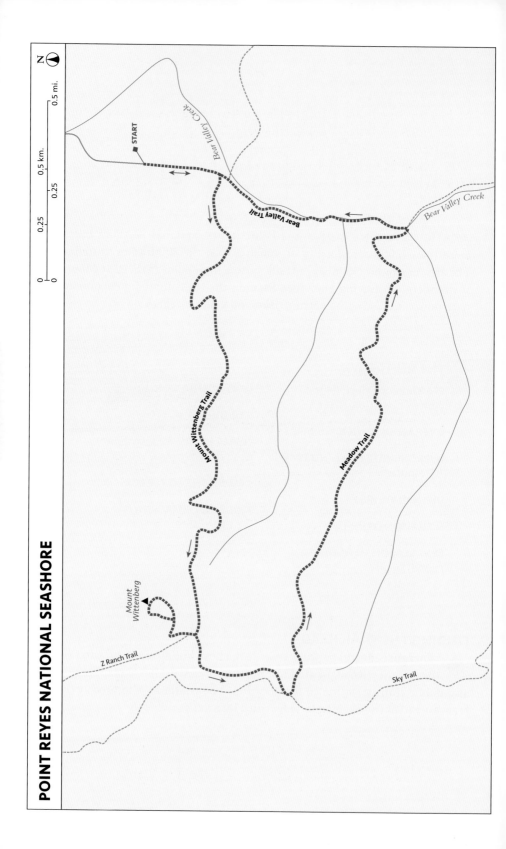

POINT REYES NATIONAL SEASHORE

N

0   0.25   0.5 km.
0   0.25   0.5 mi.

START

Bear Valley Creek

Bear Valley Trail

Bear Valley Creek

Mount Wittenberg Trail

Meadow Trail

Mount Wittenberg

Z Ranch Trail

Sky Trail

RUN DESCRIPTION

Follow the Bear Valley Trail, a wide, hard-packed gravel trail, for 0.2 mile to the junction of the Mount Wittenberg Trail on the right. This mostly singletrack trail has sections of exposed roots and rocks a well as carpets of pine needles on the upper reaches of the trail. Approximately 2 miles into the run, turn right at the junction leading to the summit, a half mile out and back. There are no views at the summit, just heavy frost. After the short out-and-back, turn right and continue on the ridge until reaching a turnoff to the Meadow Trail, which is on the left. Follow this single-track trail, which is runnable for the first three-quarters of a mile before the descending gets a bit rocky and rooted. The Meadow Trail intersects the Bear Valley Trail at the 4.5-mile point. Turn left to finish this counter-clockwise loop. There are many options to lengthen this loop by continuing on the ridge to a second (Old Pine Trail) or third (Baldy Trail) or fourth (Coast Trail) turnoff, all leading back to the Bear Valley Trail.

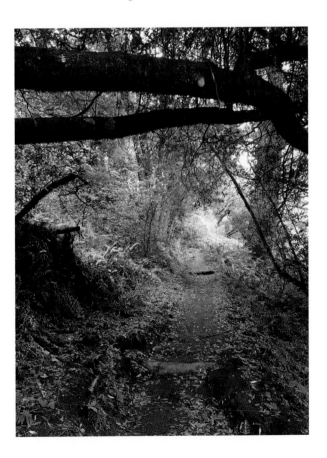

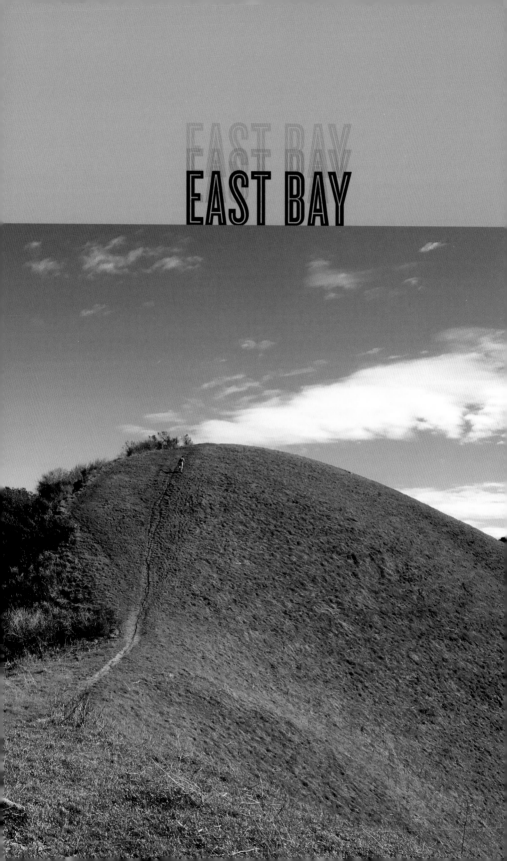

EAST BAY

WILDCAT CANYON REGIONAL PARK

LOCATED WITHIN THE CITY LIMITS of Richmond in Contra Costa County, Wildcat Canyon Regional Park offers 25 miles of trails within its 2,429 acres in the East Bay Regional Parks District. The park extends from the Tilden Nature Area above the Berkeley hills in the south to historic Alvarado Park at the north end in Richmond.

THE RUNDOWN

START: Alvarado Park; elevation 360 feet

OVERALL DISTANCE: 5.7-mile loop from parking lot

APPROXIMATE RUNNING TIME: 80 minutes

DIFFICULTY: Blue. A few steep climbs. Nothing technical.

ELEVATION GAIN: 1,150 feet

BEST SEASON TO RUN: Avoid the trail during or after heavy rains due to muddy sections complete with cow patties and open terrain with little to no shade.

DOG FRIENDLY: Off-leash areas in open space (although sections in the park—Tilden Nature Area—are off-limits to dogs)

PARKING: Free parking at the trailhead, with overflow parking on street in adjacent neighborhood

OTHER USERS: Equestrians. Cyclists are permitted in sections of the park, but not in the Tilden Nature Area.

CELL PHONE COVERAGE: Very good

MORE INFORMATION: www.ebparks.org/parks/wildcat#trailmap

EAST BAY

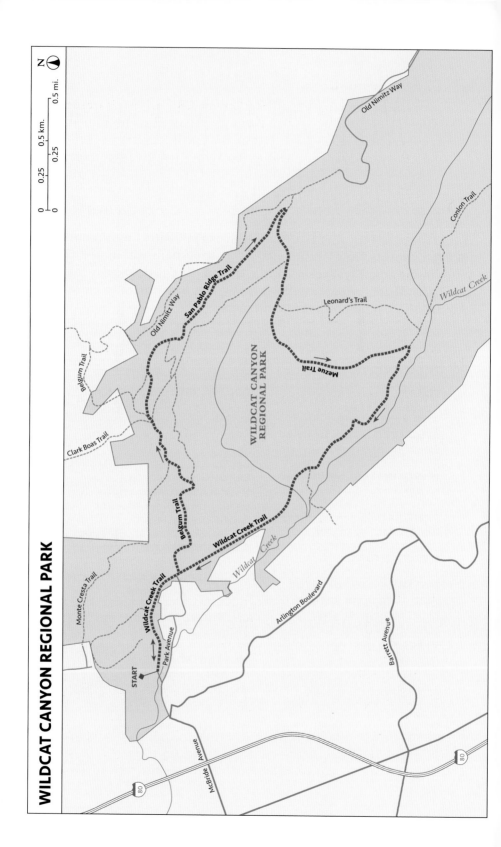

WILDCAT CANYON REGIONAL PARK

N

0   0.25   0.5 km.
0   0.25   0.5 mi.

Old Nimitz Way

Conlon Trail

Wildcat Creek

Leonard's Trail

Mezue Trail

San Pablo Ridge Trail

Old Nimitz Way

Belgum Trail

Clark Boas Trail

WILDCAT CANYON
REGIONAL PARK

Belgum Trail

Wildcat Creek Trail

Wildcat Creek

Monte Cresta Trail

Wildcat Creek Trail

START

Park Avenue

Arlington Boulevard

Barrett Avenue

McBride Avenue

80

80

FINDING THE TRAILHEAD

The Alvarado trailhead in Wildcat Canyon Regional Park is accessed from North Richmond and Pinole by taking I-80 west to the McBryde exit, turning left at the bottom of the ramp and heading onto McBryde Avenue. Follow McBryde to the second stop sign, where stone

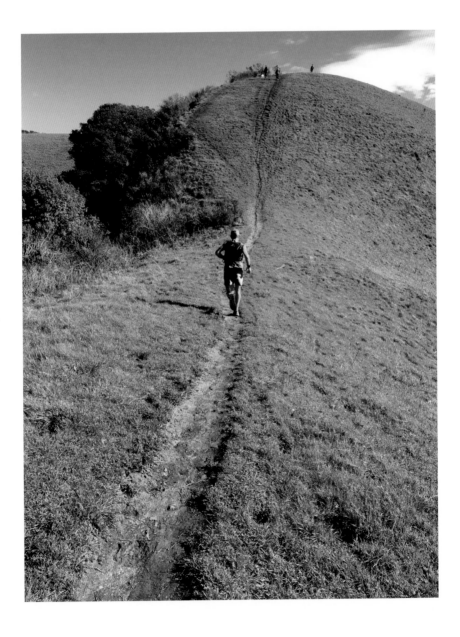

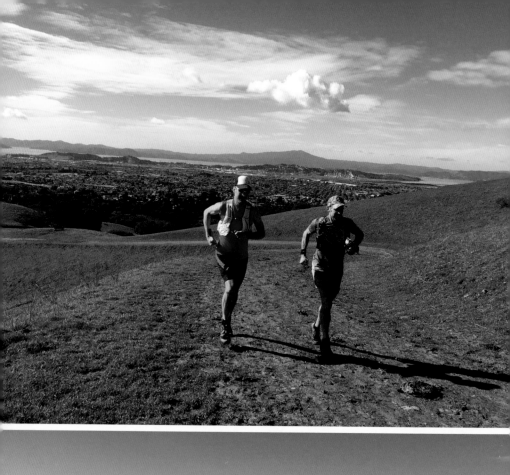

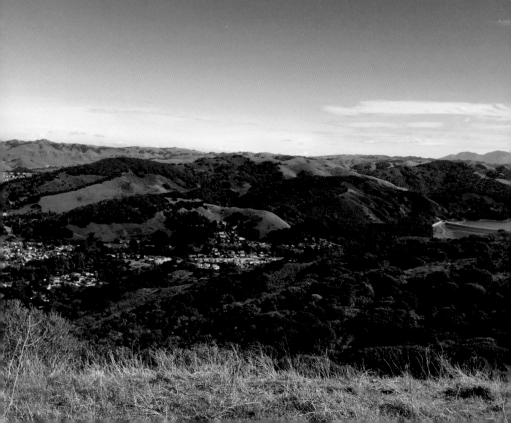

pillars to the north mark the entrance to Alvarado Park. Follow the paved parking lot approximately a quarter mile uphill to the trailhead.

RUN DESCRIPTION

From the trailhead marker follow the Wildcat Creek Trail for approximately 0.5 mile to the intersection and take the San Pablo Ridge Trail, which forks to the left. At just under 3 miles, turn right to join the Mezue Trail, which intersects back with Wildcat Creek Trail at the 4-mile point. Follow it back to the parking lot. This route connects to numerous trails covering a vast area offering abundant ascending/descending and flat and rolling terrain. Running this loop clockwise has some very steep climbs. Trails are primarily fire roads, with a smattering of singletrack. The views are expansive and outstanding, including San Francisco in the distance as well as the Richmond and Golden Gate Bridges and Mount Diablo. There is a paved section of slightly more than 1 mile that may help you decide whether to run clockwise (paved section is mostly downhill) or counterclockwise (paved section is mostly uphill).

EAST BAY

BRIONES REGIONAL PARK

A TRAIL-RUNNING TRIP TO THE BAY AREA is not complete without a visit to one of the sixty-five parks in the East Bay Regional Park District. With more than 1,250 miles of trails, there is sure to be terrain to your liking.

Briones Regional Park is just one of the many venues sure to pique a trail runner's interest. Amidst the rolling hills and seasonally lush green pastures covering some 6,200 acres, there are several trailhead access points providing relatively flat running as well as quality ascending and descending on a mixture of fire roads and singletrack trails.

There are five locations through which to enter the park; the most developed are the Bear Creek Staging Area at 16 Bear Creek Road in Lafayette and Alhambra Creek Valley Staging Area off Reliez Valley Road near Martinez.

ABRIGO VALLEY TRAIL TO MOTT PEAK LOOP

THE RUNDOWN

START: Bear Creek Staging Area; elevation 697 feet

OVERALL DISTANCE: 3.2-mile clockwise loop

APPROXIMATE RUNNING TIME: 40 minutes

DIFFICULTY: Green. Easy, but a bit of climbing.

ELEVATION GAIN: 607 feet

BEST SEASON TO RUN: Dry. During periods of heavy moisture, many of the trails are a sloppy mess with the combination of mud and cow patties.

DOG FRIENDLY: Signage indicates which areas require dogs to be on a leash.

PARKING: Day use fee, with a small additional fee for dogs.

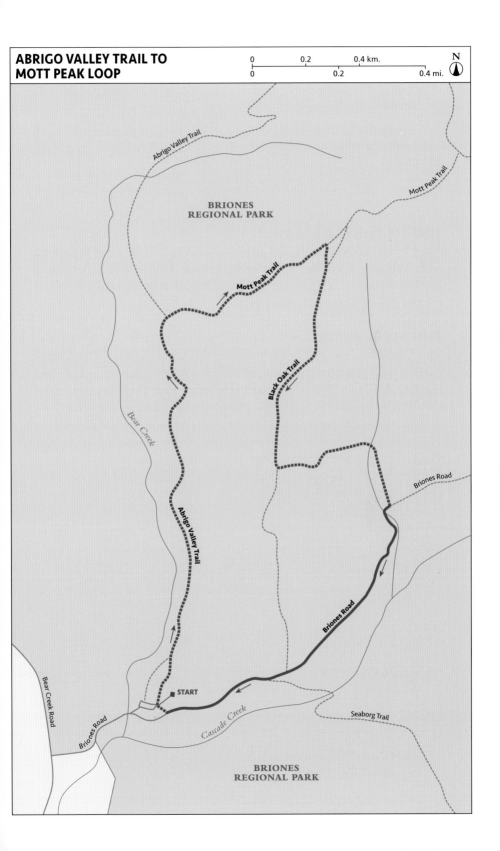

0   0.2   0.4 km.

0   0.2   0.4 mi.

N

Abrigo Valley Trail

Mott Peak Trail

BRIONES
REGIONAL PARK

Mott Peak Trail

Black Oak Trail

Bear Creek

Abrigo Valley Trail

Briones Road

Briones Road

Bear Creek Road

Briones Road

START

Cascade Creek

Seaborg Trail

BRIONES
REGIONAL PARK

Annual passes are available for purchase.

OTHER USERS: Equestrians and cyclists allowed on designated trails

CELL PHONE COVERAGE: Good

MORE INFORMATION: www .ebparks.org/parks/briones/

FINDING THE TRAILHEAD

From San Francisco take I-80 east to CA 24 east. Take exit 9 to Camino Pablo in Orinda and follow to Bear Creek Road at the intersection of San Pablo Dam Road. Continue to Briones Valley Road and the parking lot for this staging area and trailhead.

RUN DESCRIPTION

The route has good signage and starts on the Abrigo Valley Trail, a hard-packed, wide path that leads to a dirt fire road. After about 1 mile turn right on the Mott Peak Trail. Continue to the Black Oak Trail, intersecting to the right. Following a short climb, the route continues downhill and connects with the Old Briones Road. Turn right and return to the parking lot. The route is very open with wide vistas from the higher points on the trail. Cows graze unfettered, a welcome sight, although cow patties are prevalent. The final three-quarters of a mile of the route is paved (the Old Briones Road).

DIABLO VIEW TO ALHAMBRA CREEK TRAIL

THE RUNDOWN

START: Alhambra Creek Valley Staging Area; elevation 376 feet

OVERALL DISTANCE: 2.5-mile clockwise loop

APPROXIMATE RUNNING TIME: 30 minutes

DIFFICULTY: Green. Easy, but a bit of climbing.

ELEVATION GAIN: 574 feet

BEST SEASON TO RUN: Dry. During periods of heavy moisture, the dirt trails become a bit sloppy.

DOG FRIENDLY: Signage indicates which areas require dogs to be on a leash.

PARKING: Day use fee, with a small additional fee for dogs. Annual passes are available for purchase.

OTHER USERS: Equestrian friendly, with bikes allowed on designated trails

CELL PHONE COVERAGE: Good

MORE INFORMATION: www .ebparks.org/parks/briones/

FINDING THE TRAILHEAD

From Orinda take CA 24 east to Pleasant Hill Road. Head north to Reliez Valley Road and continue on to the park entrance at Brockwood Drive on the left. Follow to the staging area and parking lot. The trailhead is at the gate on the south side of the parking lot.

RUN DESCRIPTION

The route has good signage and starts just beyond the gate on a dirt fire road, the Diablo View Trail. Continue on to the Spengler Trail intersection, turning right after about 1 mile. At the next intersection, at the 1.5-mile point, reach the Alhambra Valley Trail to the right and continue back to the parking lot. The initial climb affords fantastic views and wide-open

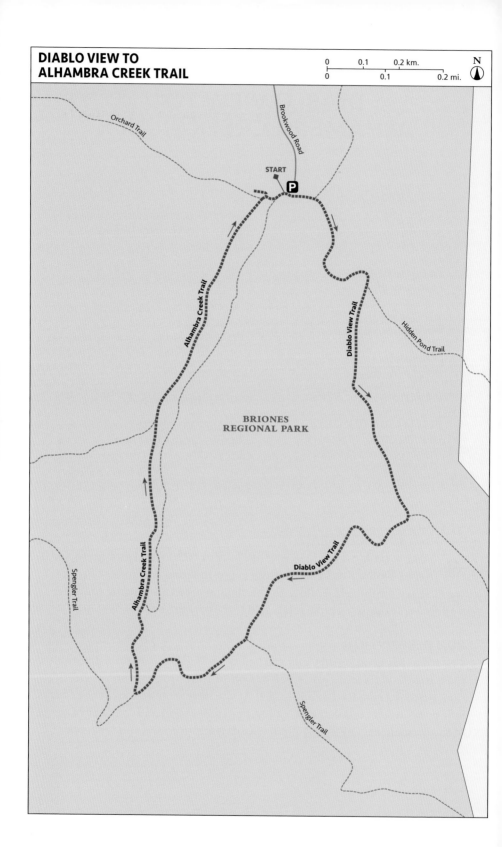

0   0.1   0.2 km.

0   0.1   0.2 mi.

N

Orchard Trail

Brookwood Road

START

P

Alhambra Creek Trail

Diablo View Trail

Hidden Pond Trail

BRIONES
REGIONAL PARK

Spengler Trail

Alhambra Creek Trail

Diablo View Trail

Spengler Trail

spaces. A portion of the route is on singletrack trails, and sections of the trail meander through the forest. Some sections can be muddy during the rainy season, but the runoff is better on this side of the park, as there are more hard-packed and gravel-laden trails.

SHELL RIDGE OPEN SPACE

THE 31 MILES OF TRAILS IN SHELL RIDGE OPEN SPACE provide a variety of choices. There are wide dirt pathways, open grassy areas, singletrack trails, and quality ascents and descents in a very serene locale. Affording amazing 360-degree views of the East Bay from the higher points along the ridge, this area is magical.

Trails are well signed but can be confusing with the many trail connectors and intersections. **Note:** It is recommended to take a map along on runs in this area.

SUGARLOAF–SHELL RIDGE TRAIL TO RIDGE TOP TRAIL WITH SECTIONS OF SULFUR CREEK TRAIL AND COSTANOAN TRAIL

THE RUNDOWN

START: Rockspring Place trailhead; elevation 366 feet

OVERALL DISTANCE: 6.2-mile keyhole route with out-and-backs for vistas

APPROXIMATE RUNNING TIME: 80 minutes

DIFFICULTY: Blue. Some decent climbs.

ELEVATION GAIN: 1,344 feet

BEST SEASON TO RUN: Dry. During periods of heavy moisture, the wider trails are a sloppy and very slippery mess with the combination of mud and cow patties.

DOG FRIENDLY: Some off-leash areas; some areas not dog friendly

PARKING: On-street parking is free near the trailhead and is in a residential neighborhood.

SUGARLOAF–SHELL RIDGE TRAIL

0   0.25   0.5 km.
0   0.25   0.5 mi.

N

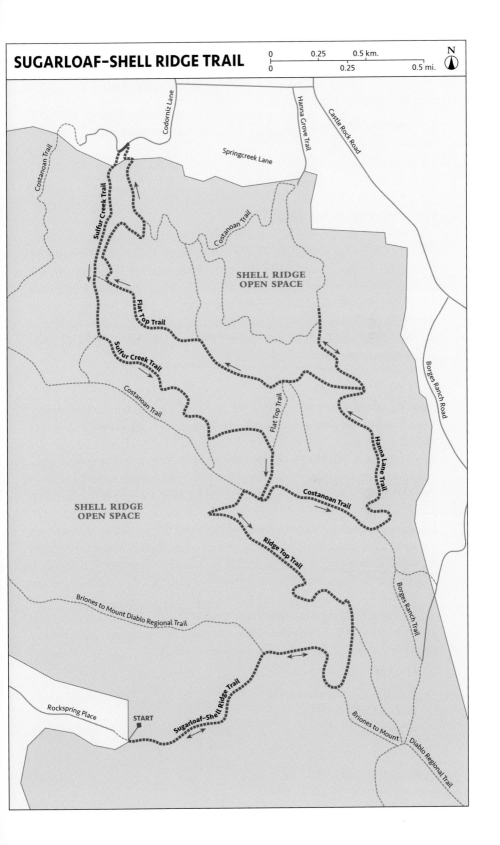

OTHER USERS: Equestrians, bicyclists on designated trails

CELL PHONE COVERAGE: Good

MORE INFORMATION: www.ci.walnut-creek.ca .us/Home/Components/ FacilityDirectory/Facility Directory/10/664

FINDING THE TRAILHEAD

From San Francisco follow I-80 east toward Emeryville and continue to CA 24 east to South Main Street in Walnut Creek. Take exit 45A from I-680 south and continue to Rudgear Road, heading east, and turn left on San Miguel Drive. Continue to Mountain View Boulevard and turn right; follow to Walnut Boulevard and turn right and finally left on Rockspring Place. This road is a dead end to the trailhead. Park in this residential neighborhood and note the gate and trailhead signage between two houses at the end of the road.

RUN DESCRIPTION

Starting at the Rockspring Place trailhead on the Sugarloaf–Shell Ridge Trail, head uphill on the wide pathway. Reach the Ridge Top Trail, and at just under 1.5 miles, turn right on the Costanoan Trail. This trail continues downhill to become the Hanna Lane Trail. Follow for a short out-and-back and return for a right turn onto the Flat Top Trail, which actually ascends and descends in spite of its name. Following a spur trail from the Flat Top Trail, which becomes the Costanoan Trail at about 3 miles into the run, return on a short keyhole route after reaching the border to the park on a spur of the Costanoan Trail. At approximately 3.8 miles, start ascending on Sulfur Creek Trail for the next mile and meet back with the Ridge Top Trail. Continue to ascend for a quarter mile and then descend back to the trailhead.

This route has a mixture of wide dirt paths and singletrack trails in open meadows as well as in forested sections. From the high points the views of the valley below and nearby cities are outstanding.

Trail Surfaces: Mud, Snow, and Ice

No San Francisco trail-running guide worth its salt would neglect to address mud running, given its prominence. The best way to deal with mud on the trail is to enjoy it, and to get as dirty as possible early in the run so you won't worry about it thereafter. Soft mud enables a lower-impact run, especially on the descents, where mud provides a great surface for slowing the pace without stressing joints.

To avoid slipping, it may help to shorten your stride, run more upright than normal, and keep your elbows more angled for lateral balance. If you begin to slip, try to relax and control the recovery so as not to overreact and fall in the opposite direction.

If water is running down the trail, the best bet is to run where water is moving most rapidly because that surface will probably be the firmest. A faster current tends to remove most of the sticky sediment, leaving behind gravel and rock. Although the runner will get wet, the likelihood of getting bogged down in muddier trail borders is markedly decreased. This technique is also friendlier to the trail because of the lower environmental impact.

From an environmental standpoint, resist the temptation to run alongside the trail in an effort to avoid getting muddy. Submitting to the temptation leads to wider trails; and if everyone did it, pathways would soon be major thruways instead of singletrack trails. Typical Bay Area weather causes muddy trails, and depending on the sensitivity of the specific trail system, it may be advisable to avoid certain trails until they have a chance to dry.

Although they are uncommon for San Francisco, snow and ice do occasionally hit the trails. Running with confidence is more important on snow and ice than on any other surface. Although most runners are hesitant on snow and ice, the trick is to try to tuck away that insecurity, take a deep breath, relax, and run with a sense of command. Admittedly, snow and ice—being inanimate elements—cannot read minds; however, they manage to wreak havoc on runners who fear them. Fearful runners run with tense form, lean back, and often resort to jerky, sudden movements in an attempt to adapt to the slick surface. That is just the opposite of what works best for running on slick snow or ice.

The best form for snow and ice running is a slight forward lean that distributes the body's weight evenly across the foot as it hits the slippery surface. Fluid, steady movement is less likely to cause a loss of traction. In the event of slipping on snow or ice, the best response is to relax and to try to let your body flow with a calculated response. Do not try and stop or brake, as that will just cause you to slide out and fall. Resist the impulse to tense up or make a sudden movement to counter the slipping, which all too often leads to slipping even more. Instead, relax and breathe steadily. Even if slipping on snow and ice does lead to a fall, being relaxed will reduce the likelihood of injury. Besides, one of the best benefits of snow is that it cushions the impact.

Snowshoeing and running with traction devices or ice spikes are alternatives that make trails accessible no matter how much it snows or whether the trails are covered by ice. The snow's forgiving compressibility and the impact absorption from snowshoes' increased surface area make it feel as though you are running on wood-chip-lined trails.

DON EDWARDS SAN FRANCISCO BAY NATIONAL WILDLIFE REFUGE

A HIDDEN GEM IDEAL FOR THE NOVICE TRAIL RUNNER, this area is peaceful and serene in spite of its close proximity to Dunbarton Bridge and the hectic pace of the city. The trails connect via a pedestrian overpass to Coyote Hills Regional Park, one of the East Bay's regional parks, sporting 978 acres and 12.5 miles of trails providing a step up to more challenging trails.

THE RUNDOWN

START: Don Edwards Visitor Center; elevation 48 feet

OVERALL DISTANCE: 2.3 miles

APPROXIMATE RUNNING TIME: 25 minutes

DIFFICULTY: Green

ELEVATION GAIN: 183 feet

BEST SEASON TO RUN: Year-round. Trails have great runoff and absorption.

DOG FRIENDLY: Leashed dogs on designated trails

PARKING: Free

OTHER USERS: Bikes on designated trails

CELL PHONE COVERAGE: Good

MORE INFORMATION: www .fws.gov/refuge/don_edwards_ san_francisco_bay/

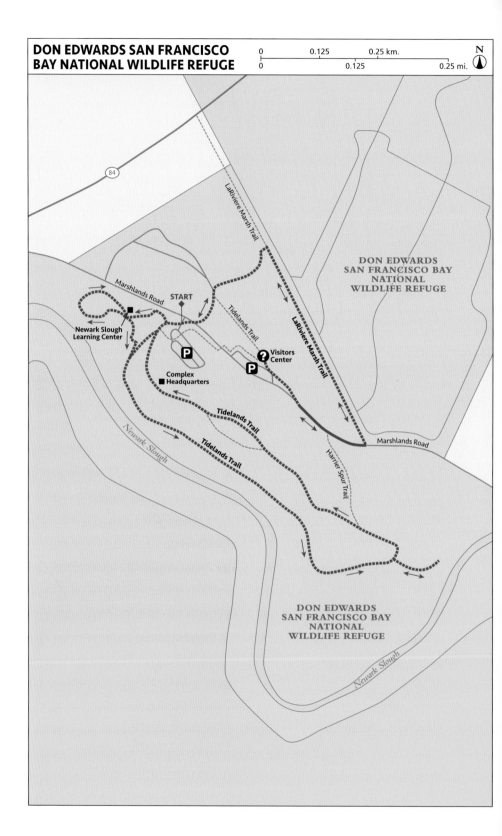

FINDING THE TRAILHEAD

From South San Francisco follow US 101 south to CA 84 east over the Dunbarton Bridge. Take exit 36 to Thornton Avenue and follow it south to Marshlands Road. Turn right on Marshlands Road and continue to the parking lot near the visitor center.

RUN DESCRIPTION

Starting at the Marshlands Road trailhead, follow the Tidelands Trail as it loops around the Newark Slough. After about 1 mile turn left to make a short loop around the Newark Slough Learning Center and then cross over Marshlands Road to connect with the LaRiviere Marsh Trail. Turn right at the intersection and continue to Marshlands Road and back to the parking lot. This short circuit provides a great feel for the area. The terrain is relatively flat with some gentle grades. Vistas abound, geckos are ever present on the trail, and marshland grasses mix with California poppies.

MISSION PEAK REGIONAL PRESERVE

COMPRISING 3,000 ACRES, this is yet another glorious spot in the East Bay Regional Park system, which butts up to the 6,859-acre Sunol Regional Wilderness via the Ohlone Wilderness Trail, a 3.59-mile connector (permit required for access), for even more enjoyable trails. Park at either Ohlone College or the more popular and crowded Stanford Avenue access lot. The trails from these two parking areas connect for longer routes. The Ohlone College parking area is located approximately 2 miles from the Stanford Avenue access lot.

THE RUNDOWN

START: Stanford Avenue parking lot; elevation 386 feet

OVERALL DISTANCE: 3.8-mile counterclockwise loop

APPROXIMATE RUNNING TIME: 50 minutes

DIFFICULTY: Blue due to elevation changes

ELEVATION GAIN: 1,195 feet

BEST SEASON TO RUN: Can be muddy during times of significant rainfall

DOG FRIENDLY: Leashed dogs

PARKING: Free

OTHER USERS: Equestrian and bicyclist friendly

CELL PHONE COVERAGE: Good

MORE INFORMATION: www.ebparks.org/parks/mission

FINDING THE TRAILHEAD

 From South San Francisco follow US 101 south to CA 92 east, crossing the San Mateo Bridge to I-880 south. Follow to CA 262 north/Mis-

MISSION PEAK REGIONAL PRESERVE

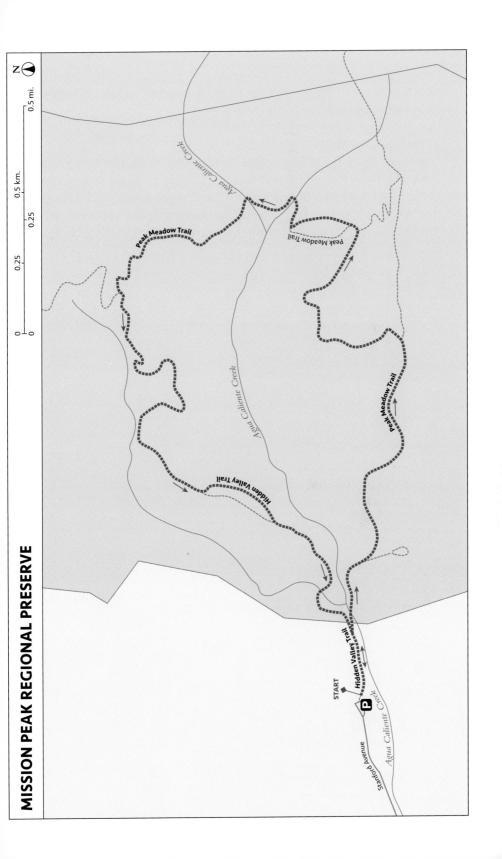

sion Boulevard in Fremont. Turn right on Stanford Avenue, which is a dead end, to the parking lot for the trailhead.

RUN DESCRIPTION

Start the run on the Hidden Valley Trail; at the fork take the right onto Peak Meadow Trail, which will make this a counterclockwise loop intersecting back with the Hidden Valley Trail at approximately 2.3 miles into the run. Enjoy picture-perfect views to the west on the upper reaches of the Peak Meadow Trail, and relish in the downhill back to the parking lot.

FREMONT OLDER OPEN SPACE PRESERVE AND STEVENS CREEK COUNTY PARK

THIS AREA PROVIDES TWO ENTIRELY DIFFERENT trail-running experiences. The open space area is a 739-acre preserve with wide trails and quality ascents, while the county park provides 1,077 acres with over 6 miles of singletrack trails with sections of technical terrain. Runs in this area provide a mixed bag, a virtual olio of trail running.

THE RUNDOWN

START: Stevens Canyon Road parking area; elevation 550 feet

OVERALL DISTANCE: 6.4-mile clockwise loop

APPROXIMATE RUNNING TIME: 75 minutes

DIFFICULTY: Blue, due to ascending and switchbacks on singletrack sections. A mixed bag of terrain underfoot makes this a great destination.

ELEVATION GAIN: 1,175 feet

BEST SEASON TO RUN: Year-round. Trails have great runoff and absorption.

DOG FRIENDLY: Leashed dogs are allowed on all trails.

PARKING: Free on-street parking adjacent to trailhead by the dam, or paid parking in the designated lot off Stevens Canyon Road

OTHER USERS: Equestrians and mountain bikers on designated trails in the open space; equestrians and mountain bikers on all trails in the park

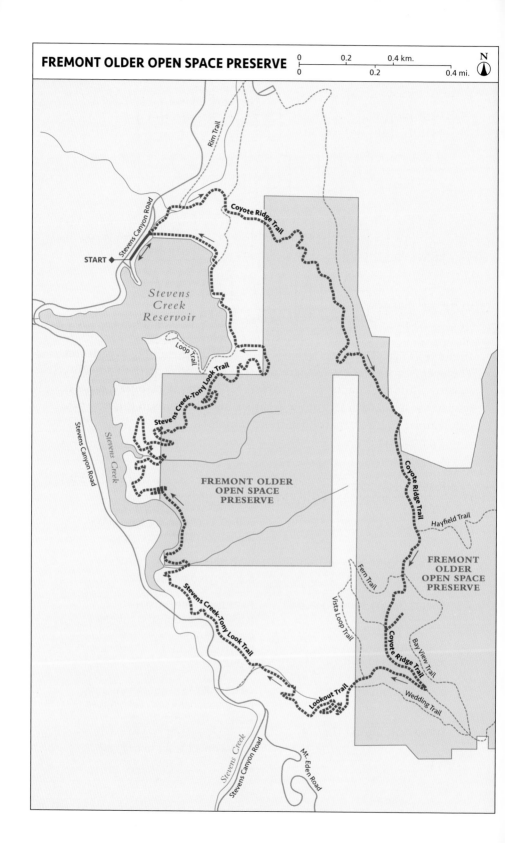

FREMONT OLDER OPEN SPACE PRESERVE

0   0.2   0.4 km.
0   0.2   0.4 mi.

N

Rim Trail

Coyote Ridge Trail

Stevens Canyon Road

START

Stevens Creek Reservoir

Loop Trail

Stevens Creek-Tony Look Trail

Stevens Canyon Road

Stevens Creek

FREMONT OLDER OPEN SPACE PRESERVE

Coyote Ridge Trail

Hayfield Trail

FREMONT OLDER OPEN SPACE PRESERVE

Fern Trail

Vista Loop Trail

Stevens Creek-Tony Look Trail

Coyote Ridge Trail

Bay View Trail

Lookout Trail

Wedding Trail

Stevens Creek

Stevens Canyon Road

Mt. Eden Road

CELL PHONE COVERAGE: Good

MORE INFORMATION: www
.openspace.org/preserves/

fremont-older; www.sccgov
.org/sites/parks/parkfinder/
Pages/StevensCreek.aspx

FINDING THE TRAILHEAD

From South San Francisco take US 101 south to I-280 south. Exit to Foothill Boulevard, heading south to Stevens Canyon Road in Cupertino. There is off-street parking on the road near Stevens Creek by the dam.

RUN DESCRIPTION

Run parallel to the road, heading north to reach the Rim Trail located on the north side of the dam. After 0.3 mile connect to the Coyote Ridge Trail to gain the high point in the preserve at Maisie's Peak after approximately 2 miles. This is a very short out-and-back from the Coyote Ridge Trail. After enjoying the view, follow Coyote Ridge downhill for a short distance to connect with the Vista Loop Trail, which forks to the right and reaches the Lookout Trail, where singletrack terrain prevails for the remainder of this clockwise loop. The Lookout Trail at times runs parallel to Stevens Canyon Road and along the eastern edge of Stevens Creek, where the name changes to the Tony Look Trail. When you reach the northern side of the dam, return south to the parking area on Stevens Canyon Road.

EAST BAY

MOUNT DIABLO STATE PARK

WITH APPROXIMATELY 20,000 ACRES and its namesake high point of 3,849 feet, the Mount Diablo State Park provides numerous trail-running opportunities on its 520 miles of trails. There are two entrance stations, one at Northgate Road in Walnut Creek, the other at Diablo Road in Danville. Runs can include a venture to the summit, where on a clear day one can see nearly 200 miles in the distance, or a variety of routes near the base. Trails are very well marked.

THE RUNDOWN

START: El Molino Road in Clayton; elevation 442 feet

OVERALL DISTANCE: 6.3 miles

APPROXIMATE RUNNING TIME: 70 minutes

DIFFICULTY: Blue

ELEVATION GAIN: 984 feet

BEST SEASON TO RUN: Year-round, but some creek crossing and slick spots in heavy rain

DOG FRIENDLY: No

PARKING: Daily use fee, but there are options to park free along residential streets.

OTHER USERS: Equestrians. Mountain bikes are permitted on fire roads and three designated trails.

CELL PHONE COVERAGE: Good

MORE INFORMATION: www .parks.ca.gov/?page_id=517

FINDING THE TRAILHEAD

From Clayton Road in Clayton, turn right on Marsh Creek Road and then right on El Molino Road for on-street parking across from 196 El Molina. This route starts approximately 1 mile outside the park

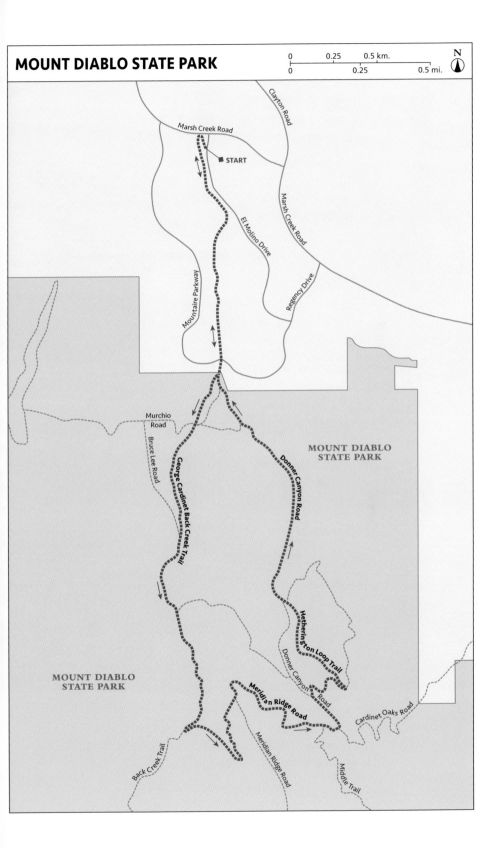

0   0.25   0.5 km.

0   0.25   0.5 mi.

N

Clayton Road

Marsh Creek Road

START

Marsh Creek Road

El Molino Drive

Regency Drive

Mountaire Parkway

Murchio Road

Bruce Lee Road

George Cardinet Back Creek Trail

Donner Canyon Road

MOUNT DIABLO STATE PARK

Hetherington Loop Trail

Donner Canyon Road

Meridian Ridge Road

MOUNT DIABLO STATE PARK

Cardinet Oaks Road

Back Creek Trail

Meridian Ridge Road

Middle Trail

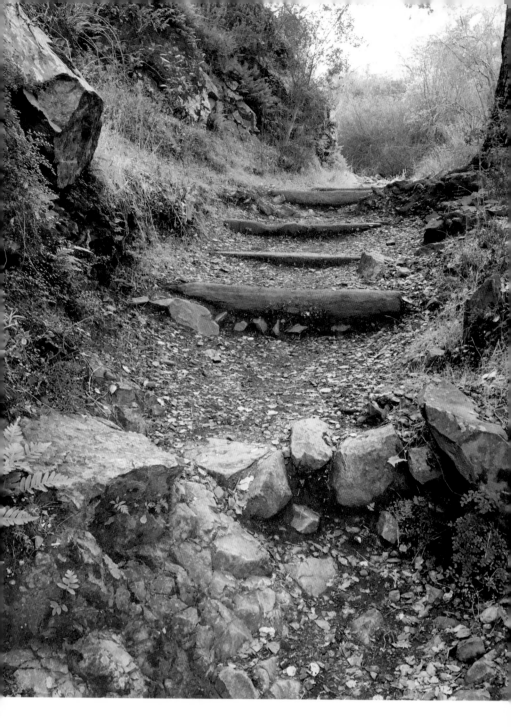

entrance, starting on the sidewalk parallel to El Molino, followed by a left on Marsh Creek Road and then a quick left on Mt. Wilson Way. The singletrack trail is reached within 50 feet on the left.

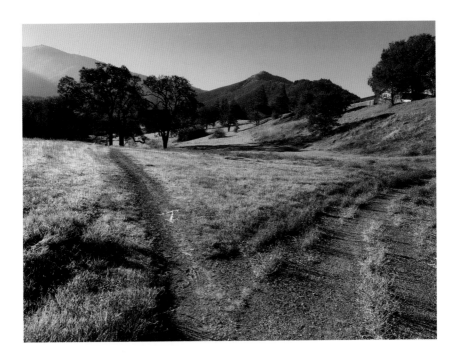

RUN DESCRIPTION

Follow the singletrack trail to the gate entrance to Mount Diablo State Park. Leashed dogs are allowed only until the park property. After passing through the gate, head uphill on the right on singletrack designated Back Creek Trail. The next 2 miles is a mix of fire road and singletrack and crosses a few creek beds that are mostly dry in the summer but may get your feet wet. The trail goes in and out of shaded forest and serves up views of Mount Diablo to the soutn and the town of Clayton to the north. The climb is substantial, reaching the high point of just over 1,400 feet in 3 miles. At the junction head downhill on a fire road (starting as Meridian Ridge Road and becoming Donner Canyon Road) for approximately three-quarters of a mile and turn back onto singletrack Hetherington Loop Trail, complete with switchbacks. After 4 miles cross a footbridge and return to the Donner Canyon Road. Follow this back to the park entrance gate and return on the singletrack to the start point for this keyhole counterclockwise loop. The Dirt Dogs, a trail-running club in the East Bay, frequents the park on its weekly runs.

REDWOOD REGIONAL PARK

A PRIZE IN THE EAST BAY REGIONAL PARKS DISTRICT, Redwood Regional Park is located in the hills east of Oakland. Boasting the largest remaining natural stand of coast redwood found in the East Bay, this park has 1,830 acres with nearly 40 miles of singletrack trails and fire roads abutting open space properties for additional trail-running opportunities. The Joaquin Miller Park and Huckleberry Botanic Regional Preserve are to the west and north, respectively, and to the south is the Anthony Chabot Regional Park. With numerous trail access points, some of which do not require a park fee, the opportunities for a full day on the trails are endless. Trails are well marked at most junctions, but carrying a map is suggested to ensure you are on the correct route.

THE RUNDOWN

START: Big Bear Staging Area; elevation 638 feet

OVERALL DISTANCE: 3 miles

APPROXIMATE RUNNING TIME: 40 minutes

DIFFICULTY: Blue

ELEVATION GAIN: 573 feet

BEST SEASON TO RUN: Year-round

DOG FRIENDLY: Leashed dogs

PARKING: Free at this staging area, with spaces for about ten cars

OTHER USERS: Equestrians and mountain bikers on designated trails

CELL PHONE COVERAGE: Poor

MORE INFORMATION: www.ebparks.org/parks/redwood

REDWOOD REGIONAL PARK

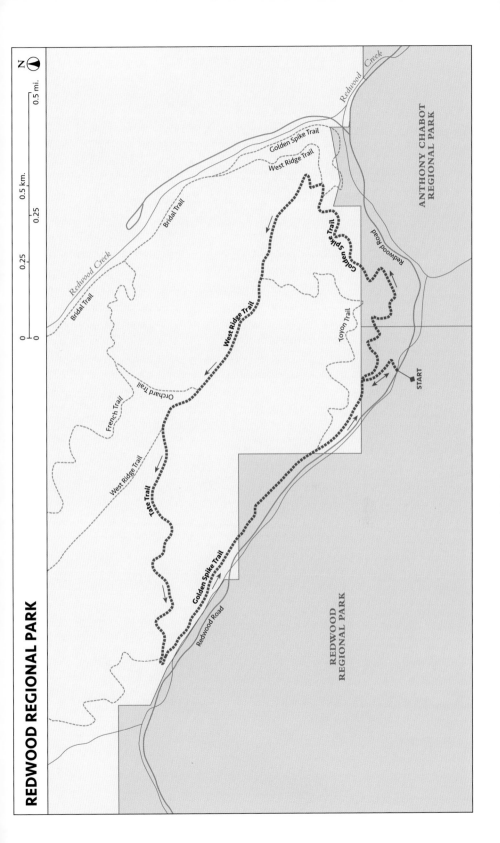

N

0   0.25   0.5 km.

0   0.25   0.5 mi.

Redwood Creek

Bridal Trail

Bridal Trail

West Ridge Trail

Golden Spike Trail

West Ridge Trail

Golden Spike Trail

French Trail

Orchard Trail

West Ridge Trail

Tate Trail

Toyon Trail

Golden Spike Trail

Redwood Road

Redwood Road

Redwood Creek

START

REDWOOD
REGIONAL PARK

ANTHONY CHABOT
REGIONAL PARK

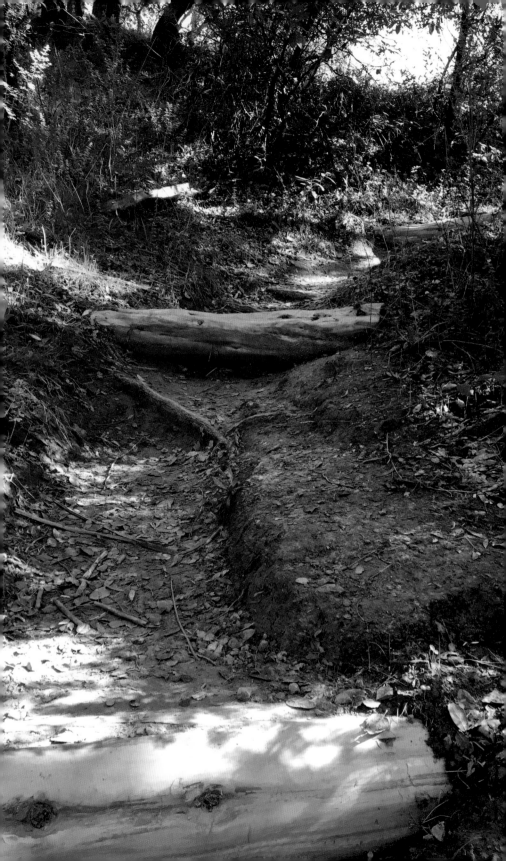

FINDING THE TRAILHEAD

This short loop starts at the Big Bear Staging Area on Redwood Road, located approximately 3 miles from the intersection of Skyline Boulevard in Oakland. **Note:** Redwood Road is a popular biking route; mind the speed limit and watch for cyclists. The parking area is on the right side of the road and is marked.

RUN DESCRIPTION

Cross Redwood Road to start this route. Head uphill and turn right on the marked Golden Spike Trail, which is singletrack. Continue uphill for much of the next mile and reach the West Ridge Trail junction and turn left on this fire road. Continue uphill for another half mile, and the road flattens out a bit. Follow to the junction of the Tate Trail (no bikes on this trail) at just under 1.5 miles. This mostly downhill singletrack reaches the junction of the Golden Spike Trail at about the 2-mile mark. Turn left and return on this rolling singletrack to a right-hand turn for Redwood Road. Return to the start point of this counterclockwise loop.

EAST BAY

COYOTE HILLS REGIONAL PARK

ANOTHER GEM IN THE EAST BAY REGIONAL PARKS DISTRICT, this nearly 1,000-acre park is mostly exposed, providing views of the Dunbarton Bridge, San Francisco Bay, and Foster City to the west and Mission and Sunol Peaks to the east from the upper reaches of the trail system. A mix of singletrack, boardwalks, fire roads, and paved pathways provides visitors with a variety of trail-running opportunities. The paved Bayview Trail connects with 12 additional miles of trail along the south levee of the Alameda Creek Trail to reach the Don Edwards San Francisco Bay National Wildlife Refuge.

THE RUNDOWN

START: Patterson Ranch Road parking lot; elevation 22 feet

OVERALL DISTANCE: 3.1 miles

APPROXIMATE RUNNING TIME: 40 minutes

DIFFICULTY: Green (based on terrain); blue (based on climbing)

ELEVATION GAIN: 448 feet

BEST SEASON TO RUN: Year-round

DOG FRIENDLY: Dogs on leash

PARKING: Day use fee, with a small additional fee for dogs

OTHER USERS: Mountain bikes on paved roads

CELL PHONE COVERAGE: Good

MORE INFORMATION: www .ebparks.org/parks/coyote_ hills#features

FINDING THE TRAILHEAD

 From I-880 in Fremont take CA 84 west; exit at Paseo Padre Parkway, turn right, and drive north about 1 mile to the entrance on

COYOTE HILLS REGIONAL PARK

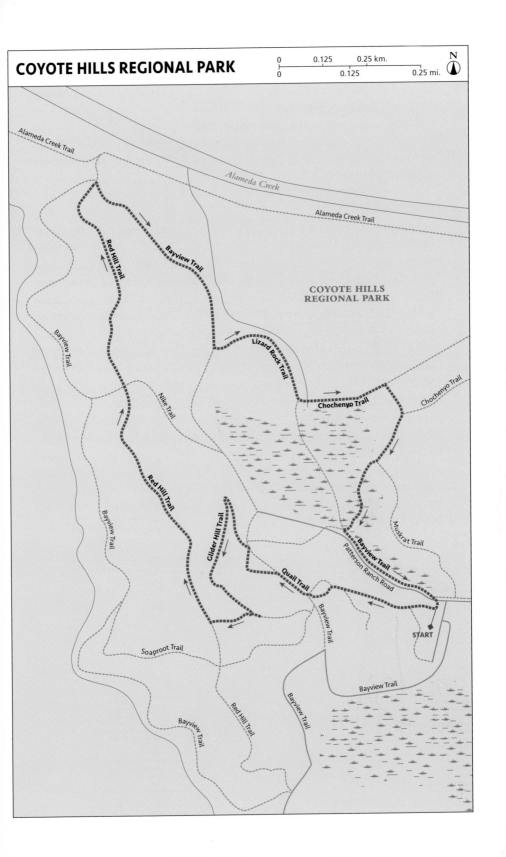

0   0.125   0.25 km.
0   0.125   0.25 mi.

N

Alameda Creek Trail

Alameda Creek

Alameda Creek Trail

Red Hill Trail

Bayview Trail

Bayview Trail

COYOTE HILLS
REGIONAL PARK

Lizard Rock Trail

Nike Trail

Chochenyo Trail

Chochenyo Trail

Red Hill Trail

Bayview Trail

Glider Hill Trail

Bayview Trail

Muskrat Trail

Patterson Ranch Road

Quail Trail

Bayview Trail

START

Soaproot Trail

Bayview Trail

Red Hill Trail

Bayview Trail

Bayview Trail

Patterson Ranch Road. (Although there is limited free parking on Patterson Ranch Road at the corner of Paseo Padre Parkway, it is over a mile to reach the trails within the park.) After passing through the toll gate on Patterson Ranch Road, continue to the first parking lot—the Quarry Staging Area—on the left side of the road. The start of the route is just north of the parking lot on the Muskrat Trail.

RUN DESCRIPTION

The start of this route is on an uphill, wide, dirt and gravel path. Continue uphill for about 0.3 mile to the junction of the Quail Trail. Turn right on this fire road and continue until reaching the junction of the Glider Hill Trail. This singletrack trail is mostly uphill and reaches a lookout point at 233 feet in elevation after less than 1 mile. Continue to the junction of the Red Hill Trail and follow it north (to the right). There is a steep descent, followed by a steep, short ascent with sweeping 360-degree vistas. Continue on Red Hill Trail, which descends to the junction of the paved Bayview Trail, which for much of its length offers a dirt shoulder. Turn left on the Lizard Rock Trail and, after less than a quarter mile of weaving through the marshland, connect to the Chochenyo Trail, a wide gravel path. Cross over a boardwalk back to the Bayview Trail (or at the junction take the Muskrat Trail to reach the starting point of the route). Turn left on the roadway and finish back at the staging area after a quarter mile. Although a short loop, this route offers plenty of variety with some lung-busting climbing, speedy descending, and flat running on a mix of surfaces. Bring sunscreen and linger after the run with a pair of binoculars to view the birds in the wetlands.

BUYING NEW TRAIL-RUNNING SHOES

Begin by looking at the wear and tear of your old, "spent" shoes. Are the soles worn in certain parts and not in others? Wear patterns provide evidence of overpronation or -supination. By looking at wet footprints left after a shower, bath, or swim and comparing your prints with others, you can determine relative arch height and forefoot width. Armed with those particular "foot notes," a trail runner is better able to shop for shoes at a local specialty running store, in a catalog, or from an online vendor and ask an expert salesperson for a recommendation. It is best to go to a running specialty store where a foot specialist can perform a gait analysis with a videotaped treadmill or other test.

When shopping for trail shoes, wear the same kind of socks worn for running. Similarly, those who use orthotics should bring the devices to ensure shoes fit once the orthotic is inserted. Also, it is best to shop immediately or soon after a run, when your feet are most likely to be swollen. Ultrarunners should err on the side of buying a half to a whole size larger than normal to accommodate foot swelling.

Be wary of buying a new model or style of shoes from a catalog or website. Just because a trail runner has liked a brand of shoe does not mean that the runner will be happy with another model or style from the same manufacturer. Similarly, just because a trail runner enjoys a particular shoe model does not guarantee that the next iteration with the same model name will fit or perform in a similar manner. Shoe manufacturers are always tweaking their lines in an effort to better the product, and all too often those "improvements" leave the runner with a shoe that goes by the same name but has an entirely different feel, fit, or performance. When in doubt, buy from a local retailer, especially if you can test-drive the shoes on a treadmill or in the parking lot.

LAKE CHABOT REGIONAL PARK

WITH 20 MILES OF TRAILS, there is something for everyone's running palate in this East Bay regional park located in Castro Valley. This park connects to an additional 70 miles of trails in the adjoining Anthony Chabot Regional Park. In addition to trail running, boating, fishing, and picnicking are all activities available in the park.

THE RUNDOWN

START: Lake Chabot Marina parking lot; elevation 270 feet

OVERALL DISTANCE: 4.6 miles

APPROXIMATE RUNNING TIME: 45 minutes

DIFFICULTY: Green

ELEVATION GAIN: 624 feet

BEST SEASON TO RUN: Year-round, although some of the dirt sections in the forest can be muddy during and after heavy rains.

DOG FRIENDLY: Leashed dogs

PARKING: For parking in the marina lot, there is a fee (and a small additional fee for dogs). An East Bay Regional Park annual pass is available. Free parking on street. Can be extremely busy on the weekends.

OTHER USERS: Bicyclists and equestrians on designated trails

CELL PHONE COVERAGE: Good

MORE INFORMATION: www .ebparks.org/parks/lake_ chabot

FINDING THE TRAILHEAD

Although there are many access points to the park, this featured route is accessed via the Lake Chabot Marina parking lot, which is located west of Lake Chabot Road in Castro Valley. From I-580 west, take the

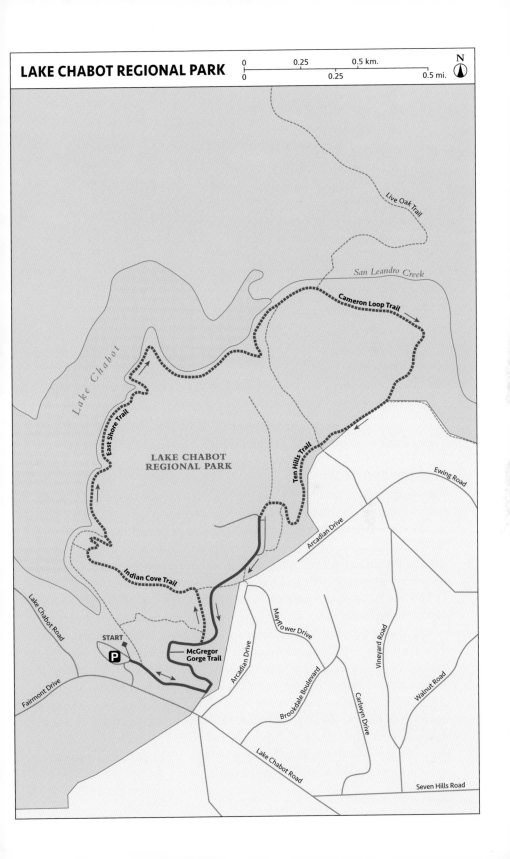

0   0.25   0.5 km.

0   0.25   0.5 mi.

N

Live Oak Trail

San Leandro Creek

Cameron Loop Trail

Lake Chabot

East Shore Trail

Ten Hills Trail

LAKE CHABOT
REGIONAL PARK

Ewing Road

Arcadian Drive

Indian Cove Trail

Lake Chabot Road

START

P

McGregor
Gorge Trail

Arcadian Drive

Mayflower Drive

Vineyard Road

Fairmont Drive

Brookdale Boulevard

Carlwyn Drive

Walnut Road

Lake Chabot Road

Seven Hills Road

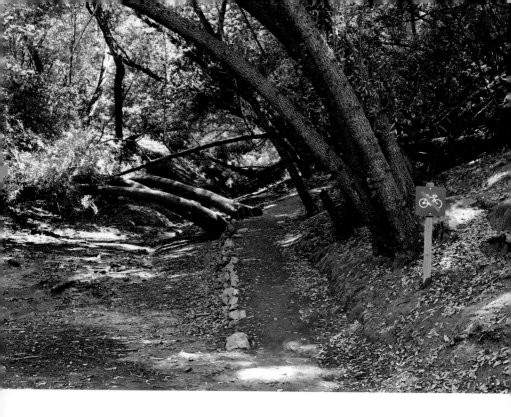

Strobridge Avenue exit toward Hayward. Follow Stanton Avenue to Castro Valley Boulevard; turn right, and then turn left on Lake Chabot Road.

RUN DESCRIPTION

Start in the gravel parking lot located northeast of the tollbooth, heading east. Proceed to the McGregor Gorge Trail, which is accessed after crossing the road. This doubletrack trail is hard-packed gravel and dirt running parallel to the road. After half a mile cross the road and start climbing to join the Indian Cove Trail. Continue on a short climb and then a descent on a dirt and grassy path and follow for another half mile to East Shore Trail. Turn right on this paved bike trail (which has a small dirt and gravel path running adjacent for much of the way) and continue for the next mile to join the wider, dirt-laden Cameron Loop Trail, which joins the Ten Hills Trail, or complete as a full loop on the Cameron Loop Trail returning to the East Shore Trail. If you continue on the Ten Hills Trail, follow it southward and rejoin the McGregor Gorge Trail just beyond the Regional Parks Police/Fire Headquarters and Nike Classroom. Follow the McGregor Gorge Trail back to the starting point. There are numerous trail options in the park, from singletrack to fire roads and paved paths. A bridge off the Cameron Loop Trail connects to the west side of the park and numerous trail options to make a full day on the trails.

GARIN/DRY CREEK PIONEER REGIONAL PARKS

WITH NEARLY 5,000 ACRES boasting 27 miles of trails (and future land acquisitions planned to increase the acreage), this East Bay Regional Parks duo offers spectacular views spanning downtown San Francisco to the San Mateo Bridge to the west and rolling hillsides to the north and east. Although the trails are not technical, focus is required, as the constant hoofprints of grazing cows chew up the trail, making divots that must be carefully navigated to avoid tripping or rolling an ankle. And if it is climbing you're after, these trails deliver. Enjoy sustained ascents, coupled with flat and rolling terrain as well as steep descents.

EAST BAY

THE RUNDOWN

START: May Road parking lot; elevation 125 feet

OVERALL DISTANCE: 5 miles

APPROXIMATE RUNNING TIME: 55 minutes

DIFFICULTY: Green (but with a lot of climbing)

ELEVATION GAIN: 1,041 feet

BEST SEASON TO RUN: Year-round, but avoid after heavy rains.

DOG FRIENDLY: Leashed or under voice control

PARKING: Free

OTHER USERS: Bikers on designated trails, equestrians

CELL PHONE COVERAGE: Good

MORE INFORMATION: www .ebparks.org/parks/garin

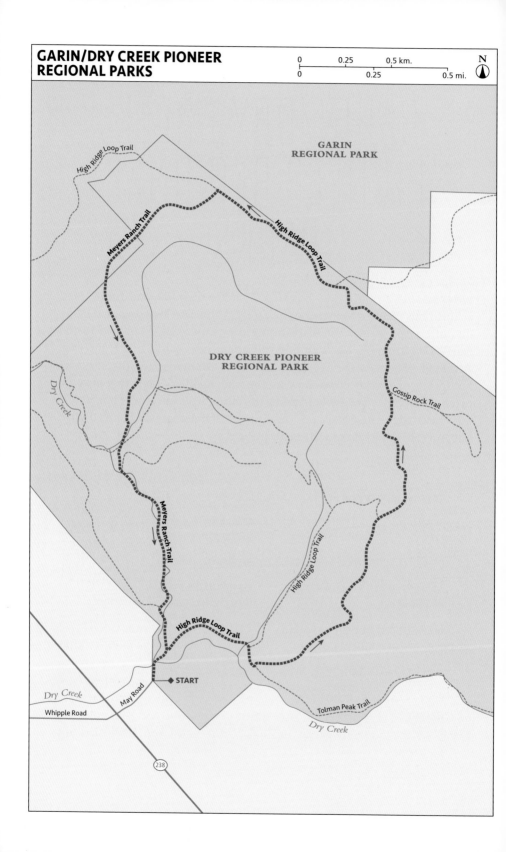

GARIN/DRY CREEK PIONEER REGIONAL PARKS

0   0.25   0.5 km.   N
0   0.25   0.5 mi.

GARIN
REGIONAL PARK

High Ridge Loop Trail

High Ridge Loop Trail

Meyers Ranch Trail

DRY CREEK PIONEER
REGIONAL PARK

Dry Creek

Gossip Rock Trail

Meyers Ranch Trail

High Ridge Loop Trail

High Ridge Loop Trail

◆ START

Dry Creek

May Road

Whipple Road

Tolman Peak Trail

Dry Creek

238

FINDING THE TRAILHEAD

There are several access points to the park, including the Garin Avenue access point, at which there is a fee to park. This route is accessed from May Road in Union City, which is a dead end located northeast of Mission Boulevard south of Hayward.

MAKE YOUR TRAIL SHOES LAST LONGER

The best way to prolong the life of trail shoes is to have several pairs and rotate them so that one pair is never used for more than a couple of consecutive runs without a rest. Using old pairs on days when the weather is "sucky" also extends the life of newer shoes that you would rather not expose to brutal conditions. Like allowing the body to have recovery days, giving shoes time off allows the midsole materials—the parts that break down the fastest—to decompress between runs.

It is a good idea to wash shoes by wiping them down to remove caked mud. Remove the insole inserts from the footbeds and insert balled-up newspaper in each footbed while the shoes dry at room temperature. If the shoes are soaked, it may be necessary to replace the newspaper once or twice.

It is best to allow shoes to dry slowly. That way they will be less likely to delaminate. Do not run the shoes through the washing machine or drier or put them in the oven, as this can damage the midsole material. Reserve your favorite trail shoes for the activity for which they were made. Do not wear them to work, for walking, or hiking, because that compresses and stresses them in ways that are not conducive to running; plus, such activities break them down prematurely.

RUN DESCRIPTION

Start the run on the May Trail, located at the northern edge of the parking lot. Follow through the gate under a forested canopy. This short section in the forest is the only shade on the route save for another short section near the 4-mile mark. Continue to the wide, packed gravel path; then turn right on the High Ridge Loop Trail and climb for the better part of 2 miles. At any junction continue left. Just before the 3-mile point, turn left to descend on Meyers Ranch Trail, a dirt and grassy singletrack. For extra mileage, instead of taking Meyers Ranch Trail, continue on the High Ridge Loop Trail, which crosses the lower reaches of the adjacent Garin Regional Park. Meyers Ranch Trail connects to the High Ridge Loop Trail at the 4.5-mile mark, where a right turn will return to the May Trail and the parking lot where the route began.

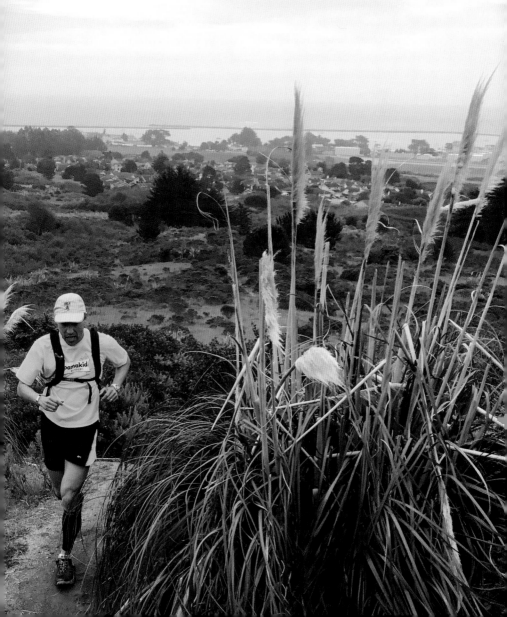

PENINSULA

SAN BRUNO MOUNTAIN STATE PARK

SAN BRUNO MOUNTAIN STATE PARK comprises 12 miles of trails within 2,416 acres. Located in northern San Mateo County, the park is adjacent to the southern boundary of San Francisco and borders the cities of Brisbane, South San Francisco, Colma, and Daly City. The mountain's ridgeline runs in an east-west configuration, with considerable slopes and elevations ranging from 250 feet to 1,314 feet at the summit. The landscape offers fantastic views of San Francisco and Central Bay Area.

SAN BRUNO MOUNTAIN SUMMIT LOOP

THE RUNDOWN

START: San Bruno Mountain State Park parking lot; elevation 700 feet

OVERALL DISTANCE: 4.6 miles

APPROXIMATE RUNNING TIME: 60 minutes

DIFFICULTY: Blue

ELEVATION GAIN: 775 feet

BEST SEASON TO RUN: Can be foggy and windy in the winter; hot, dry, and dusty in the summer. Poppies bloom in springtime, along with poison oak.

DOG FRIENDLY: No

PARKING: Free on-street parking, but a short walk to the trailhead. Parking at the trailhead has a fee.

OTHER USERS: Cyclists are allowed on some trails in the park.

CELL PHONE COVERAGE: Very good

MORE INFORMATION: https://parks.smcgov.org/san-bruno-mountain-park-trail; https://parks.smcgov.org/summit-loop-trail

SAN BRUNO MOUNTAIN
SUMMIT LOOP

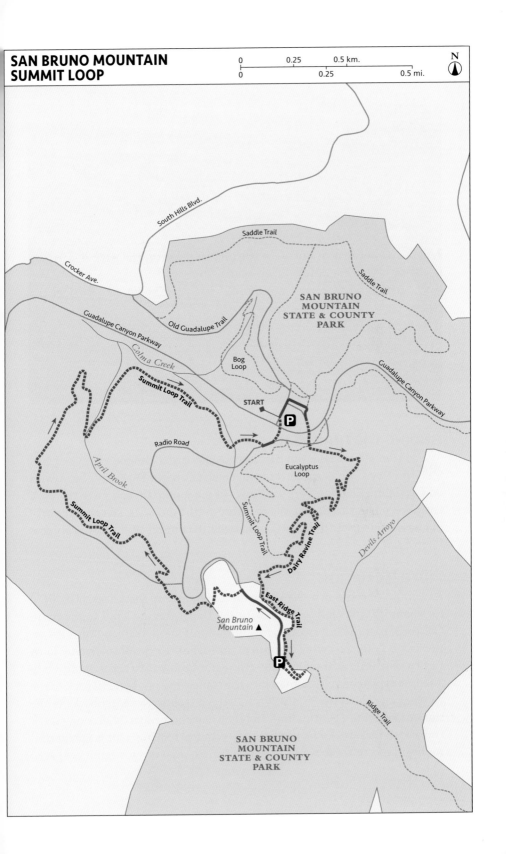

N

South Hills Blvd.

Saddle Trail

Crocker Ave.

Saddle Trail

SAN BRUNO
MOUNTAIN
STATE & COUNTY
PARK

Guadalupe Canyon Parkway

Old Guadalupe Trail

Colma Creek

Bog
Loop

Guadalupe Canyon Parkway

Summit Loop Trail

START

P

Radio Road

April Brook

Eucalyptus
Loop

Devils Arroyo

Summit Loop Trail

Summit Loop Trail

Dairy Ravine Trail

East Ridge Trail

San Bruno
Mountain ▲

P

Ridge Trail

SAN BRUNO
MOUNTAIN
STATE & COUNTY
PARK

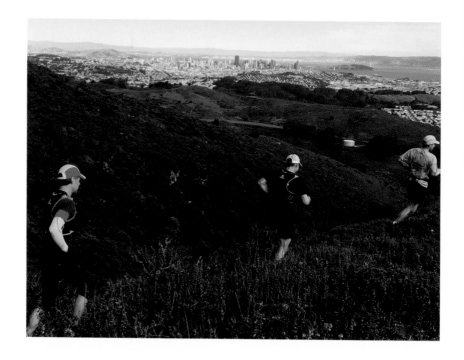

FINDING THE TRAILHEAD

From US 101 take the Bayshore Boulevard/Brisbane exit. Continue on Bayshore Boulevard to Guadalupe Canyon Parkway. Turn west on Guadalupe Canyon Parkway toward the mountain and go to the park entrance, or park free along the roadway on the shoulder. Start in the parking lot, heading south under the roadway to connect with the Eucalyptus Loop Trail.

RUN DESCRIPTION

Running the route in a clockwise direction, follow the Eucalyptus Trail for about 0.7 mile and connect with the Dairy Ravine Trail to the right. Continue past the intersection for the Summit Loop Trail and turn left on the Ridge Trail, following it uphill to the higher reaches of this route. Turn right at the intersection of Radio Road and follow it to the Summit Loop Trail, at approximately 2 miles into the route. Stay on this trail back to the parking lot. The route is mostly singletrack trail with switchbacks to the summit, offering a gentle climb and then descent, primarily on singletrack trails with some rocky sections but no technical footing. This is a great trail for beginners or those wanting to practice a tempo run for a quicker pace.

SADDLE TRAIL LOOP

THE RUNDOWN

START: Crocker Avenue, Daly City; elevation 650 feet

OVERALL DISTANCE: 3 miles

APPROXIMATE RUNNING TIME: 30 minutes

DIFFICULTY: Green

ELEVATION GAIN: 211 feet

BEST SEASON TO RUN: Year-round

DOG FRIENDLY: No

PARKING: Free on-street parking

OTHER USERS: Equestrians and cyclists are allowed on some trails in the park.

CELL PHONE COVERAGE: Very good.

MORE INFORMATION: www .parks.ca.gov/?page_id=518

FINDING THE TRAILHEAD

From Daly City follow John Daly Boulevard, turn left on Mission Street, and proceed downhill and turn right on Crocker Avenue. Park on the north side of the street along Crocker; the gate to the park is on the south side of the street. This is a residential neighborhood. Parking is also available for a fee in the park, with an entrance to the south.

RUN DESCRIPTION

Start on pavement for approximately 0.1 mile and turn left uphill on a wide, hard-packed gravel path named Saddle Trail Loop. Abundant seasonal wildflowers along with wide-open views make this an enjoyable loop on mostly rolling, smooth terrain. At the 2-mile point (which offers another access point to the park's trails from the parking lot off Guadalupe Canyon Parkway), turn left on a short half-mile loop along the Bog Trail for additional mileage if the trails are dry. As the name indicates, heavy moisture can make this mostly singletrack trail muddy in spots. Continue over a footbridge, then a short climb and gentle descent, returning on a short section of pavement to the starting point to complete the loop. Following a run at San Bruno Mountain, enjoy a meal at the Boulevard Restaurant,

SADDLE TRAIL LOOP

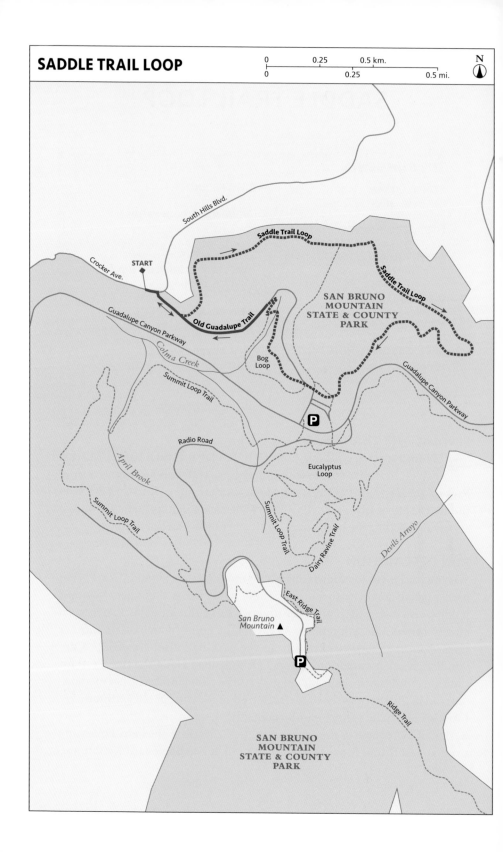

0   0.25   0.5 km.

0   0.25   0.5 mi.

N

South Hills Blvd.

Saddle Trail Loop

Crocker Ave.

START

Saddle Trail Loop

SAN BRUNO
MOUNTAIN
STATE & COUNTY
PARK

Guadalupe Canyon Parkway

Old Guadalupe Trail

Colma Creek

Bog
Loop

Summit Loop Trail

Guadalupe Canyon Parkway

P

April Brook

Radio Road

Eucalyptus
Loop

Summit Loop Trail

Summit Loop Trail

Dairy Ravine Trail

Devils Arroyo

East Ridge Trail

San Bruno
Mountain ▲

P

Ridge Trail

SAN BRUNO
MOUNTAIN
STATE & COUNTY
PARK

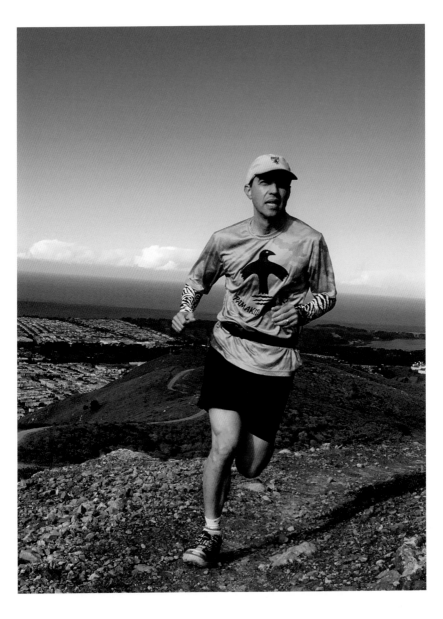

a local favorite. Since the Daly City community is predominantly Asian, especially Filipino, there are wonderful ethnic food choices as well.

SAN BRUNO MOUNTAIN RIDGE TRAIL

San Bruno Mountain is a place with great views of the Bay Area without the crowds. The Ridge Trail contains rolling slopes that eventfully descend in an eastbound direction.

THE RUNDOWN

START: End of Radio Road; elevation 1,250 feet

OVERALL DISTANCE: 4.6 miles out and back

APPROXIMATE RUNNING TIME: 25 minutes

DIFFICULTY: Moderate

ELEVATION GAIN: 1,222 feet

BEST SEASON TO RUN: Year-round

DOG FRIENDLY: No dogs allowed

PARKING: Fee to park at top of Radio Road

OTHER USERS: Mountain bikers, walkers

CELL PHONE COVERAGE: Excellent

TRAIL MARKINGS: Half-mile markers except for the 2.5-mile sign (more like 2.4). Remain on the fire road.

MORE INFORMATION: https://parks.smcgov.org/san-bruno-mountain-state-county-park

FINDING THE TRAILHEAD

From US 101 take the Bayshore Boulevard/Brisbane exit. Continue on Bayshore Boulevard to Guadalupe Canyon Parkway and turn west. After about 1.5 miles turn right into San Bruno Mountain Park. After the ranger station turn right and follow Radio Road, which will take you under the parkway and up the mountain. At the summit you will pass the transmitter towers and adjoining building. Go about 1.5 miles to the end of the road.

SAN BRUNO MOUNTAIN RIDGE TRAIL

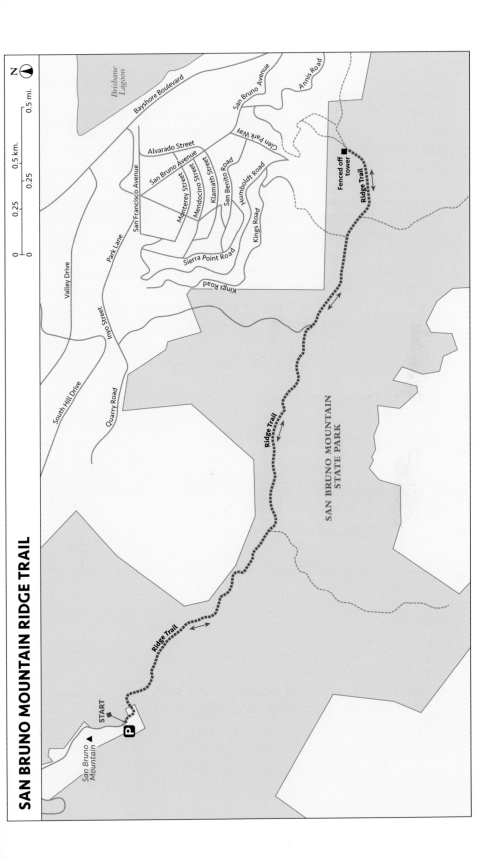

RUN DESCRIPTION

Starting at the parking lot at the end of Radio Road, enter the trail and head east. Go straight on the main trail. After about 150 yards the single-track Ridge Trail is on your left, heading north. It connects to the Summit Loop Trail. There will be half-mile signposts. Any fire roads on your right will take you down steep inclines to Hillside Road. After 1.5 miles any trails to your left will take you down steep inclines to the city of Brisbane. After 2 miles you have a choice of continuing down a 250-foot drop in a third of a mile to the 2.5-mile sign. At this point turn around. To the east is a fenced-off radio tower. The trails on either side merge at the other end. The trail continues for about a half mile before it disappears into bushes. It is not recommended that you try to find your way out. As you run, you have unobstructed views of the Bay Area and local peaks like Mount Diablo and Montara Mountain.

CROSS-TRAINING

Trail runners are often well-rounded athletes who enjoy a fine collection of outdoor endurance activities. With the changing seasons, trail runners are likely to supplement their recreational routines with Alpine and Nordic skiing; snowshoeing; mountain, road, and stationary biking; kayaking; swimming; pool running; climbing; hiking; walking; martial arts; dance; horseback riding; skating; and other pursuits. Engaging in other sports helps to balance a trail runner's training regimen, develop supporting muscles, and condition the cardio system, and throws an element of excitement and vivaciousness into the mix. Because running is not necessarily a full-body sport, integrating other activities into training helps strengthen the trunk and upper body, which might otherwise grow weak from neglect.

Skills and strengths gained from cross-training easily translate to trail running. The limbering and strengthening of muscles that comes from rock climbing; the lung capacity gained from Nordic skiing; the high-altitude training from mountaineering; the descending skills from mountain biking; the leg strength gained from snowshoeing; the muscular balance gained from swimming—all of these make for a better trail runner.

Cross-training also gives some perspective to trail running. Cross-training can be used as "active rest"—when one can feel good about not running while pursuing another discipline or developing new skills that enhance the trail-running dimension. By becoming passionate about other athletic endeavors, a trail runner is more likely to take adequate time away from running when a recovery period is necessary to recuperate from an overuse injury or to avoid overuse. Knowing that there are alternatives to running trails certainly helps during a time of injury, boredom, or burnout from running.

Cross-training is easily integrated into the trail-running routine by substituting a different discipline for a running session or two each week. These cross-training sessions should be of equivalent intensity as the running would have been, as measured by heart rate, effort, and time. For example, after a long trail run on Sunday, replace the normal 45-minute Monday recovery run with a 45-minute swim, bike, or Nordic ski session of equivalent effort.

Depending on the trail-running goals, cross-training should complement and supplement running, but not supplant it. Although cross-training is an excellent way of maintaining fitness while giving running muscles some time off, it should be thought of as active rest, in that it should not be so strenuous or depleting that one is left too exhausted to pursue trail-running training. But exercise some caution when trying a new sport, because it is easy to strain muscles that are not trained for that specific activity. It is rather disappointing to spoil your trail-running training effort because of an injury resulting from a cross-training mishap.

SWEENEY RIDGE OUT-AND-BACK

LOCATED ON THE HILLS separating the cities of Pacifica and San Bruno, the Sweeney Ridge Trail on a clear day provides outstanding views of the San Francisco Bay, San Bruno Mountain, Montara Mountain, the Pacific Ocean, and the San Francisco watershed. Spring is an ideal time to enjoy the wildflowers in bloom. The trail passes by a site connected to the Cold War years and then passes another site that commemorates the first European surveyors of the Bay Area 200 years earlier.

THE RUNDOWN

START: Skyline College parking lot; elevation 670 feet

OVERALL DISTANCE: 6.5 miles

APPROXIMATE RUNNING TIME: 80 minutes

DIFFICULTY: Blue

ELEVATION GAIN: 1,219 feet

BEST SEASON TO RUN: Year-round

DOG FRIENDLY: Dogs not allowed on Notch Trail but allowed on other trails on leash

PARKING: Free. Park users can use the Skyline College parking lot but should park in the southern end of the lot closest to the trail.

OTHER USERS: Bicyclists, walkers, and dog walkers past Notch Trail

CELL PHONE COVERAGE: Good

TRAIL MARKINGS: Excellent

MORE INFORMATION: www .nps.gov/goga/sweeney.htm

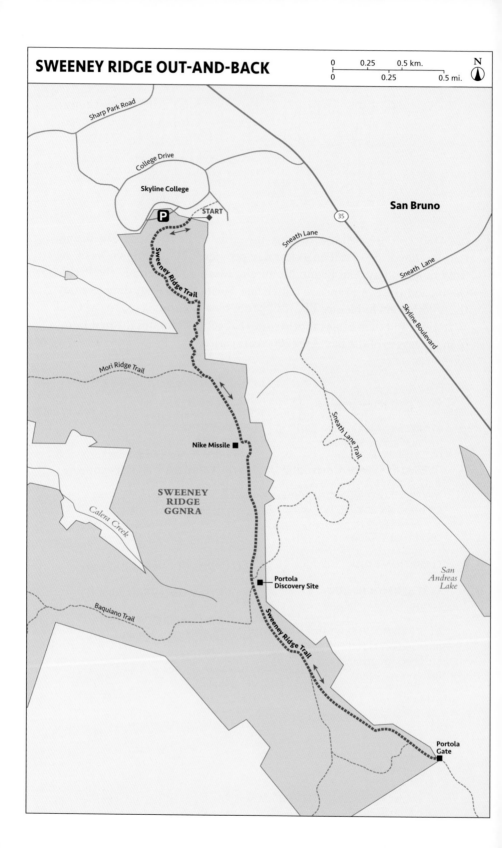

SWEENEY RIDGE OUT-AND-BACK

0   0.25   0.5 km.
0   0.25   0.5 mi.

N

Sharp Park Road

College Drive

Skyline College

P

START

San Bruno

35

Sneath Lane

Sneath Lane

Sweeney Ridge Trail

Skyline Boulevard

Mori Ridge Trail

Nike Missile ■

Sneath Lane Trail

SWEENEY
RIDGE
GGNRA

Calera Creek

San
Andreas
Lake

Portola
Discovery Site ■

Baquiano Trail

Sweeney Ridge Trail

Portola
Gate ■

FINDING THE TRAILHEAD

From CA 35/Skyline Boulevard in San Bruno, go west on College Drive. At the fork marking the entrance to Skyline College, turn left. Within 200 yards turn left into the first parking lot. After parking, walk the paved service road uphill to the maintenance facility to find the trailhead, marked by a yellow gate at the entrance. Just north of the parking lot, there is a track with water fountains.

RUN DESCRIPTION

Head up Notch Trail to reach an abandoned coast guard radio station, then continue on the Notch Trail down a ravine and then up a set of stairs. Exiting Notch Trail at the 1-mile mark, turn left and continue upward on Sweeney Trail. Just past 1.5 miles in, the route passes the former Nike missile control site, used in the Cold War, which is the highest point of the run. At this point the trail turns to pavement. Run south on the paved trail for a half mile and turn left and downhill to the entrance of Sneath Lane, where there is an outhouse. Leave the paved path and continue south on Sweeney Ridge Trail, and after a quick jaunt uphill, reach the Bay Discovery Site, which commemorates the Spanish explorer Gaspar de Portolà, who mistakenly "discovered" the San Francisco Bay in 1769 (he was looking for Monterey Bay). Head south, keeping left on the Sweeney Trail, as there will be trails to the right that go downhill to the city of Pacifica. At the locked Portola Gate, turn around for a mostly downhill run back to Skyline College.

PENINSULA

PURISIMA

PURISIMA CREEK REDWOODS OPEN SPACE PRESERVE is located on the western slopes of the Santa Cruz Mountains overlooking Half Moon Bay. The 4,711 acres feature 24 miles of developed trails complete with towering redwoods, and ferns, berries, and wildflowers in the spring and summer months. From the northern part of the preserve, you can see magnificent views of the coast and Half Moon Bay.

PURISIMA #1

THE RUNDOWN

START: North Ridge Trail trailhead on Skyline Boulevard; elevation 2,000 feet

OVERALL DISTANCE: 2.5-mile keyhole route

APPROXIMATE RUNNING TIME: 35 minutes

DIFFICULTY: Easy, with a few quick climbs, but no technical sections save an exposed root or two

ELEVATION GAIN: 384 feet

BEST SEASON TO RUN: Because the trail starts at 2,000 feet, it can be a bit cooler than the city.

DOG FRIENDLY: No

PARKING: There are limited parking spots at the trailhead (about thirty) but ample parking on the road. There is no charge for parking.

OTHER USERS: Limited access for mountain bikers and equestrians.

CELL PHONE COVERAGE: Decent signal; Verizon the best provider for the area

MORE INFORMATION: www .openspace.org/sites/default/ files/pr_purisima.pdf

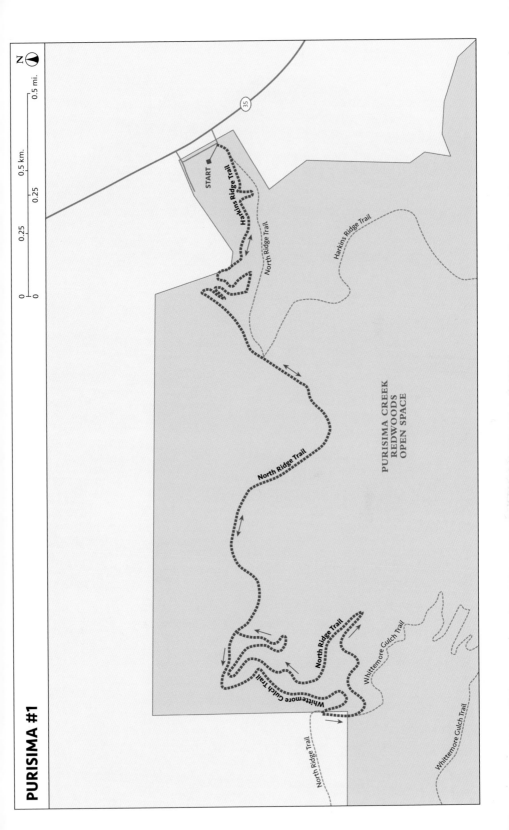

PURISIMA #1

START

Harkins Ridge Trail

North Ridge Trail

Harkins Ridge Trail

North Ridge Trail

North Ridge Trail

Whittemore Gulch Trail

North Ridge Trail

Whittemore Gulch Trail

Whittemore Gulch Trail

PURISIMA CREEK
REDWOODS
OPEN SPACE

35

N

0   0.25   0.5 km.

0   0.25   0.5 mi.

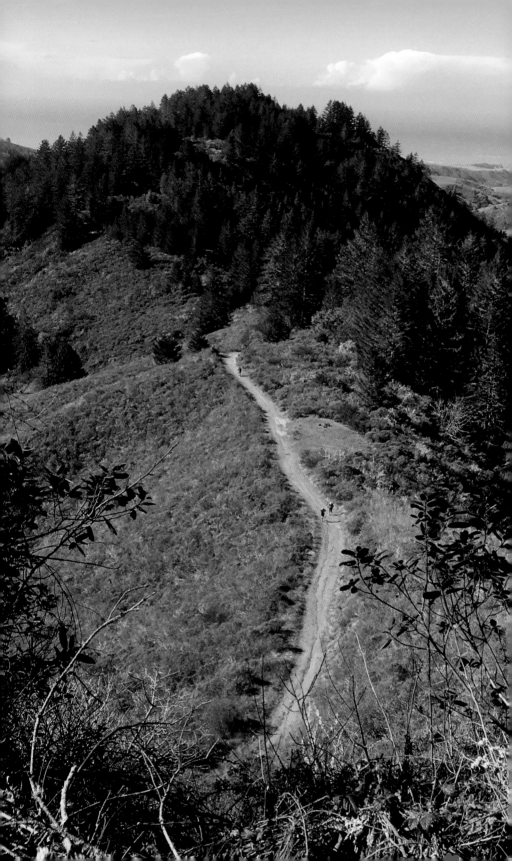

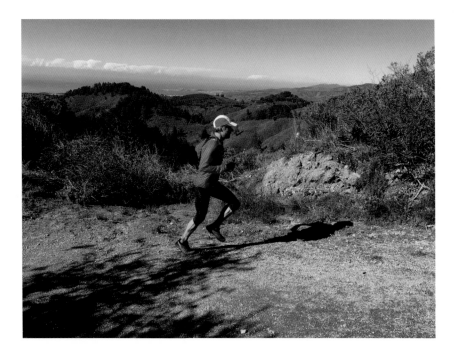

FINDING THE TRAILHEAD

From San Francisco follow US 101 south to I-280 south. Continue to exit 34 for CA 35/Skyline Boulevard. The North Ridge Trail trailhead is located on Skyline Boulevard 4.5 miles south of CA 92.

RUN DESCRIPTION

This 2.5-mile loop starts from the parking lot on the North Ridge Trail, heading south. After a level grade at the start, the route comes to rolling terrain with switchbacks through the forest, and then the trail opens to amazing vistas of Half Moon Bay. The singletrack trail captures moisture to make the surface free of dust in winter. Continue on the North Ridge Trail to the intersection of the Whittemore Gulch Trail, and turn left to return to the intersection of the North Ridge Trail and to the parking lot for this keyhole route.

PURISIMA #2

FINDING THE TRAILHEAD

From San Francisco follow US 101 south to I-280 south. Continue to exit 34 for CA 35/Skyline Boulevard. The North Ridge Trail trailhead is located on Skyline Boulevard 4.5 miles south of CA 92.

RUN DESCRIPTION

From the parking lot enjoy an out-and-back route starting on the North Ridge Trail/Harkins Ridge Trail and connecting after about 1.5 miles to the Craig Britton Trail. Continue to the intersection of the Purisima Creek Trail for the turnaround point. Enjoy second-growth redwoods and a mostly downhill run on the way out, with significant climbing on the return.

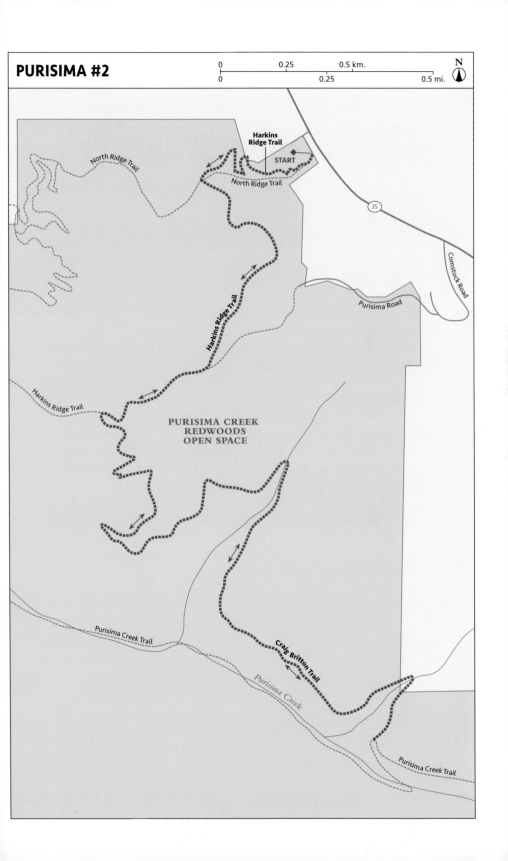

0   0.25   0.5 km.
0   0.25   0.5 mi.

N

Harkins
Ridge Trail

START

North Ridge Trail

North Ridge Trail

35

Comstock Road

Harkins Ridge Trail

Purisima Road

Harkins Ridge Trail

**PURISIMA CREEK
REDWOODS
OPEN SPACE**

Purisima Creek Trail

Craig Britton Trail

Purisima Creek

Purisima Creek Trail

TERRAIN AND TOPOGRAPHY

The terrain of the areas we've covered in this guide are quite varied. That's one of the many beauties of the San Francisco metropolitan area and its different trail-running options: There are flat runs along waterfronts and mountain runs, and you can mix them to spice things up if you'd like. We've included quite a few of each, so you may select the perfect run to match your mood, or one with specific features if you are training for a specific event.

With some of the seasonal changes, Bay Area trail runners need to be adept at running on mud, runoff, rock, and occasional snow and ice. They must know how to confront water crossings and when to avoid dangerous ones. Similarly, they must be capable of maneuvering around roots, rocks, and fallen branches; dealing with other trail obstacles; and handling wildlife confrontations.

Some of the trails in this guidebook are groomed and wide enough that they are practically dirt roads, while others are of the singletrack variety. Some allow dogs; others do not. Some turn into shoe-sucking mud when wet; others become rocky riverbeds. Still others attract local fauna during mating or nesting season. We request not only that you honor the notes about those trail sensitivities that we've provided in the guide, but also that you be very aware of the conditions and follow Leave No Trace practices in your trail running.

RANCHO SAN ANTONIO OPEN SPACE PRESERVE

WITH 24 MILES OF TRAILS and nearly 4,000 acres, this area provides many different options, with short loops on gentle grades and more-intense climbs on singletrack terrain.

THE RUNDOWN

START: Park parking area off Cristo Rey Road, Cupertino; elevation 393 feet

OVERALL DISTANCE: 2.6-mile clockwise loop

APPROXIMATE RUNNING TIME: 25 minutes

DIFFICULTY: Green

ELEVATION GAIN: 266 feet

BEST SEASON TO RUN: Year-round. Trails have great runoff and absorption.

DOG FRIENDLY: No dogs

PARKING: Free

OTHER USERS: Equestrians and mountain bikers on designated trails

CELL PHONE COVERAGE: Good

MORE INFORMATION: www.openspace.org/preserves/rancho-san-antonio

FINDING THE TRAILHEAD

From South San Francisco take US 101 south to I-280 south to Foothill Boulevard. Turn right on Cristo Rey Drive and follow it to the parking lot.

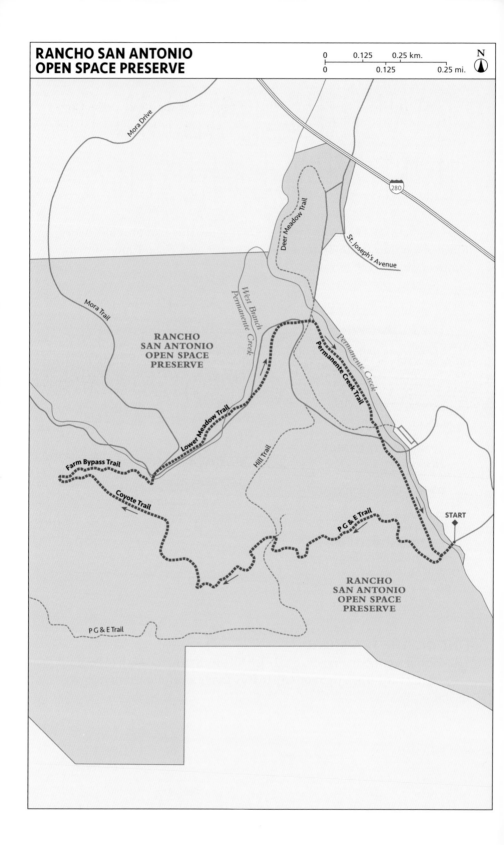

0   0.125   0.25 km.

0   0.125   0.25 mi.

N

Mora Drive

280

Deer Meadow Trail

St. Joseph's Avenue

Mora Trail

West Branch Permanente Creek

Permanente Creek

RANCHO
SAN ANTONIO
OPEN SPACE
PRESERVE

Permanente Creek Trail

Lower Meadow Trail

Hill Trail

Farm Bypass Trail

Coyote Trail

P G & E Trail

START

RANCHO
SAN ANTONIO
OPEN SPACE
PRESERVE

P G & E Trail

RUN DESCRIPTION

From the parking lot follow the trail to the left at the fork on the Coyote Trail. Continue to the intersection after approximately 1.2 miles to the Farm Bypass Trail, where you turn right and take the Lower Meadow Trail to complete this short loop.

PEARSON-ARASTRADERO OPEN SPACE

WITH 10.25 MILES OF TRAILS amid rolling savanna grassland, wildflowers in spring, and open meadows, this area has gentle grades and some challenging ascents with up to 20 percent grades in spots. Beautiful and sweeping vistas abound on this enjoyable loop, primarily on the Redtail Loop Trail.

THE RUNDOWN

START: Pearson-Arastradero Open Space parking lot; elevation 311 feet

OVERALL DISTANCE: 2.1-mile counterclockwise loop

APPROXIMATE RUNNING TIME: 20 minutes

DIFFICULTY: Green

ELEVATION GAIN: 250 feet

BEST SEASON TO RUN: Some trails (3.6 miles) in this area

can be closed seasonally if there is appreciable moisture.

DOG FRIENDLY: Dogs on leash

PARKING: Free

OTHER USERS: Equestrian and mountain bike friendly

CELL PHONE COVERAGE: Good

MORE INFORMATION: http://www.cityofpaloalto.org/gov/depts/csd/parks/preserves/arastradero/

FINDING THE TRAILHEAD

From South San Francisco follow US 101 south to I-280 south to South Page Mill Road in Palo Alto. Turn right on Arastradero Road and follow it to the parking lot.

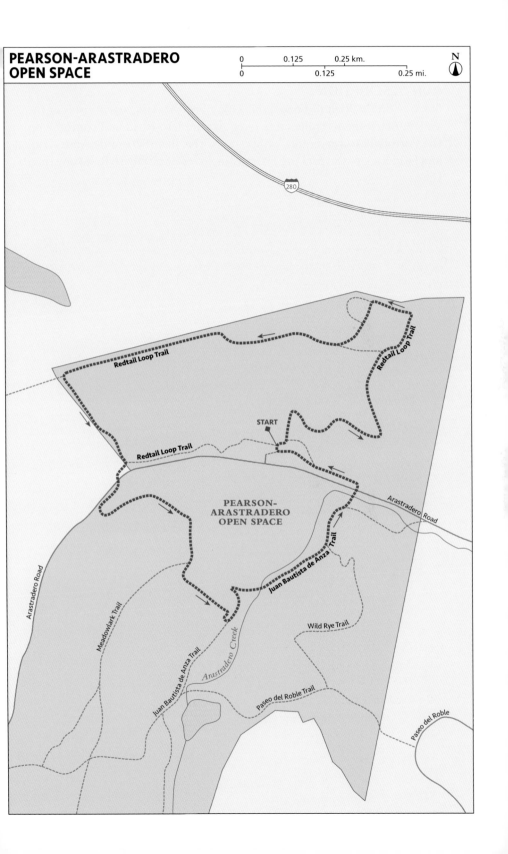

RUN DESCRIPTION

Starting on the Redtail Loop Trail, enjoy breathtaking, open vistas of the valley. After about 1 mile cross over Arastradero Road and continue on the Portola Pastures Trail. Connect with the Juan Batista de Anza Trail and head back to the parking lot, crossing over Arastradero Road one final time.

WINDY HILL OPEN SPACE

LOCATED IN SAN MATEO COUNTY, this 1,335-acre preserve features 12 miles of trails through open grassland ridges and forests of redwood, fir, and oak. The terrain is mostly smooth, alternating between fire roads and single-track trails. Although not mapped as connecting open spaces within the Portola Valley, there are dirt trails that parallel many of the main roads, providing an excellent way to travel between the open spaces in this region, including La Honda Creek Open Space to the northwest; Wunderlich Park and Huddart Park to the north; and Russian Ridge Open Space, Coal Creek Open Space Preserve, and Los Trancos Open Space Preserve to the south. There are two main parking areas, one at 555 Portola Road, the other at Skyline Boulevard 2.3 miles south of CA 84. In addition, there is some off-street parking along Skyline Boulevard.

PENINSULA

THE RUNDOWN

START: 555 Portola Road parking lot; elevation 559 feet

OVERALL DISTANCE: 7.6 miles

APPROXIMATE RUNNING TIME: 90 minutes

DIFFICULTY: Blue

ELEVATION GAIN: 1,574 feet

BEST SEASON TO RUN: Year-round

DOG FRIENDLY: Leashed pets on designated trails

PARKING: Free

OTHER USERS: Equestrians and cyclists on designated trails

CELL PHONE COVERAGE: Good

MORE INFORMATION: www .openspace.org/preserves/ windy-hill

FINDING THE TRAILHEAD

From I-280 take the Sand Hill Road exit in Portola Valley. Follow Sand Hill Road west and south; it will become Portola Road. Park at the lot on the right side of Portola Road, which accommodates twenty-five

WINDY HILL OPEN SPACE

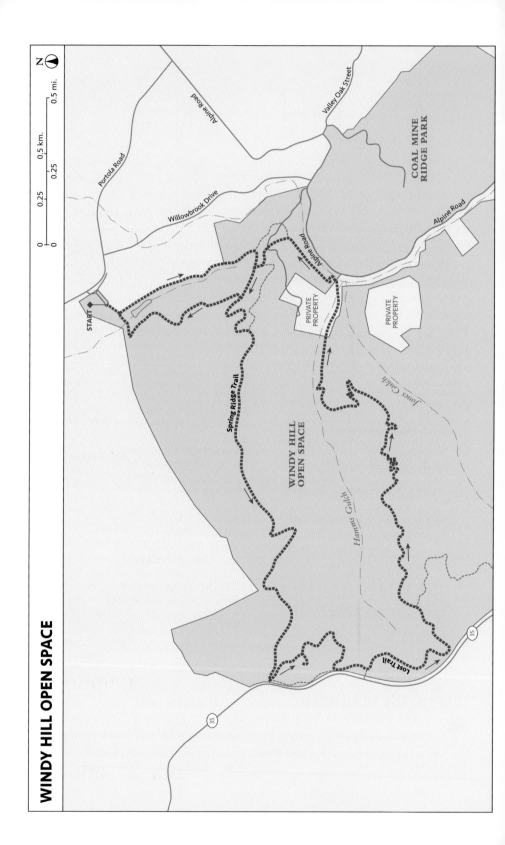

vehicles. The trailhead is on the far west side of the parking lot near the toilets.

RUN DESCRIPTION

Start on the Betsy Crowder Trail, and at the first junction turn right on the Spring Ridge Trail. At the next junction, a half mile into the run, turn

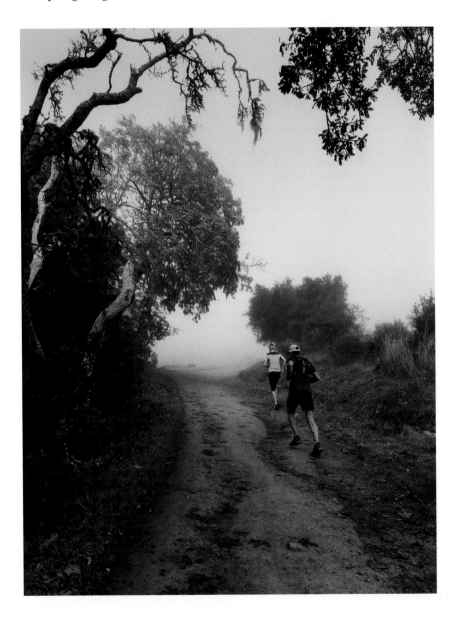

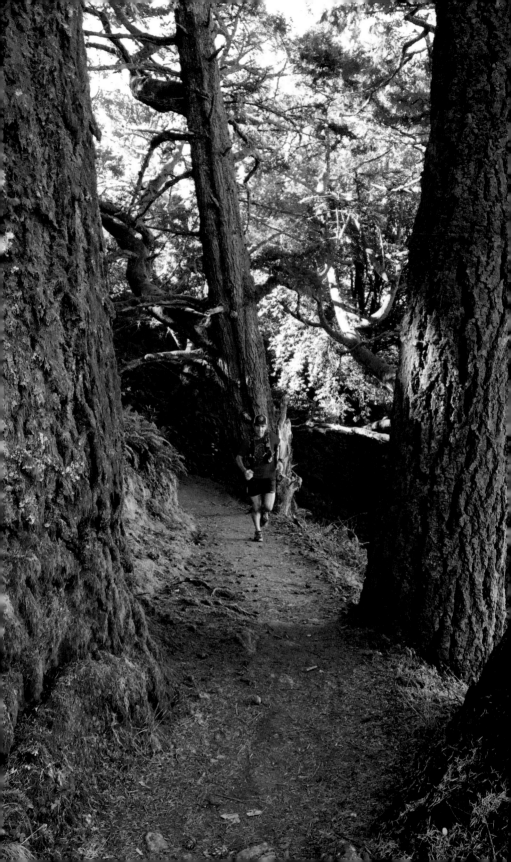

right, continuing on the Spring Ridge Trail. Follow mostly smooth trail with some long, loping switchbacks and reach Skyline Boulevard after 2.5 miles. Continue left to the summit of Windy Hill, just over 1,900 feet in elevation. Continue on the trail, descending along the ridgeline on Lost Trail. Reach the forested section of the trail 4 miles into the run and turn left on Hamms Gulch Trail, connecting to the junction of Meadow Trail at 6.5 miles. Turn left and rejoin the Spring Ridge Trail, continuing to the Betsy Crowder Trail and a finish at the parking lot.

This route provides a mixture of experiences, including open meadows with sweeping views to the north and east, glimpses of Mount Hamilton, Black Mountain to the south, as well as Mount Diablo views on a sunny day. There are long sustained climbs that lead to switchbacks in the forest for a relaxing and rolling descent. Much of the terrain in the forest is carpeted with leaves from the deciduous trees and pine needles from the coniferous vegetation overhead. There is a short section running adjacent to a creek in the forest that helps to make this run a most peaceful respite.

PENINSULA

WUNDERLICH COUNTY PARK

WITHIN THE SAN MATEO COUNTY PARK SYSTEM, there are nearly 12 miles of trails contained in the 942 acres that make up Wunderlich Park. The park is located in the midst of "horse country," and the parking lot is even placed at the foot of the historic Folger Stable. Wunderlich Park is an enjoyable area to explore on well-marked trails and dirt pathways in and out of the forest.

THE RUNDOWN

START: Parking lot off Woodside Road; elevation 515 feet

OVERALL DISTANCE: 3.1 miles

APPROXIMATE RUNNING TIME: 40 minutes

DIFFICULTY: Blue

ELEVATION GAIN: 665 feet

BEST SEASON TO RUN: Year-round

DOG FRIENDLY: No

PARKING: Free

OTHER USERS: Equestrians

CELL PHONE COVERAGE: Good

MORE INFORMATION: https:// parks.smcgov.org/wunderlich -park-trails

FINDING THE TRAILHEAD

Access the parking lot on the west side of Woodside Road/CA 84, southwest of I-280 approximately 4 miles from downtown Woodside. The trailhead is about 50 yards from the parking lot, up the paved driveway to the left of the stables.

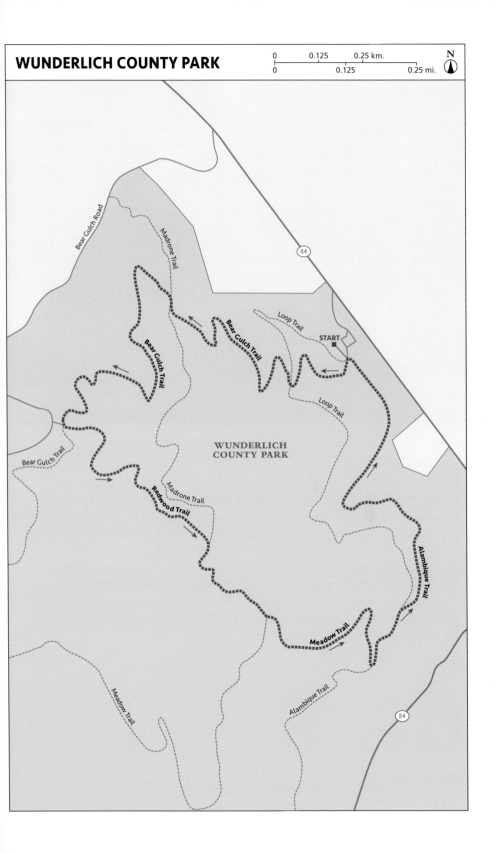

WUNDERLICH COUNTY PARK

0   0.125   0.25 km.
0   0.125   0.25 mi.

N

Bear Gulch Road

Madrone Trail

84

Loop Trail

Bear Gulch Trail

START

Bear Gulch Trail

Loop Trail

Bear Gulch Trail

WUNDERLICH
COUNTY PARK

Madrone Trail

Redwood Trail

Alambique Trail

Meadow Trail

Meadow Trail

Alambique Trail

84

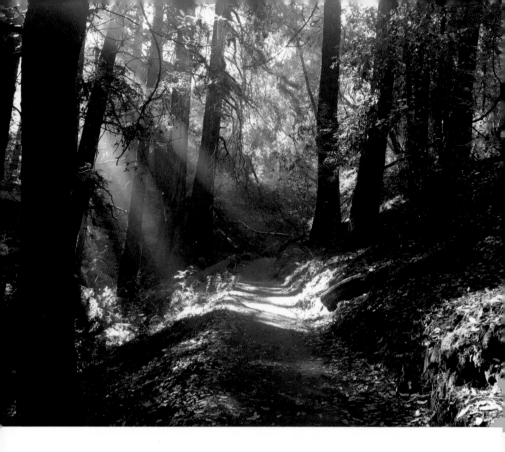

RUN DESCRIPTION

Start on the Bear Gulch Trail to ascend on switchbacks through the forest on smooth terrain and have your senses tickled by the redwood forest and eucalyptus groves through which you pass. After 1.3 miles turn left to descend on the mostly singletrack Redwood Trail, passing through Salamander Flats, where there is a moss-laden pond to the left. At the next junction, 2 miles into the run, continue on the Meadow Trail to the Alambique Trail and back to the starting point to complete this counterclockwise loop. Following the run, enjoy deli treats and snacks at Roberts Market at the intersection of Woodside Road and Canada Road or a meal at Buck's Restaurant across the street.

WaTeR CROSSINGS

Do you recall running through large puddles—or even small ponds—as a child? If so, then perhaps you mastered the technique of taking exaggerated steps with a cartoonlike form that kept you relatively dry while making everyone near you wet. That skill is invaluable, and if you don't have it down, take advantage of the dampness and warmth of spring to hone it. Go to a shallow stream, puddle, or other body of water that is not more than 6 inches deep. Think of lizards that nature programs always show running in slow motion across water. Try to duplicate that high-stepping form, and throw a little lateral kick at the end of each stride to push the water away.

For deeper water crossings, decide whether it is worth trying to stay dry. The water and air temperature, the width of the body of water, the rate of the current or flow, the availability of an alternative crossing, and the amount of time you can afford should factor into your decision. Also remember that going around water crossings, puddles, or wet areas causes erosion.

If you don't want to take the time to keep your feet dry or to change socks, consider the "easy in/easy out" alternative. Wearing highly breathable shoes with mesh uppers allows water to penetrate the shoe when confronting water crossings but also allows water to exit quickly. Water will be effectively squeegeed out of the shoe by running on dry terrain, and after a mile or two, the recent drenching will be only a faint memory. Wearing wool socks, especially ones made with merino wool that does not itch, will maintain a moderate temperature for your feet regardless of whether they are wet or dry. They will also help prevent blisters because of their temperature-regulating attributes.

HUDDART PARK OPEN SPACE

THIS 900-ACRE OPEN SPACE connects to Wunderlich Park. Bay Trail Runners (www.baytrailrunners.com) conducts an annual fall race, the Whiskey Hill Redwood Run, with a 10K and half and full marathons, that includes sections in both areas. Also in the San Mateo County Park system, Huddart Park offers more than 18 miles of trails weaving in and out of forested terrain on a mixture of singletrack and doubletrack trails.

HUDDART PARK OPEN SPACE #1

THE RUNDOWN

START: Sequoia parking lot in Huddart Park; elevation 707 feet

OVERALL DISTANCE: 3.1 miles

APPROXIMATE RUNNING TIME: 35 minutes

DIFFICULTY: Green

ELEVATION GAIN: 410 feet

BEST SEASON TO RUN: Year-round

DOG FRIENDLY: No

PARKING: Small fee, or purchase of an annual park pass

OTHER USERS: Equestrians on designated trails; cyclists on paved roads

CELL PHONE COVERAGE: Poor

MORE INFORMATION: https://parks.smcgov.org/huddart-park

FINDING THE TRAILHEAD

 From downtown Woodside head west on Woodside Road/CA 84 to King's Mountain Road. Turn right and follow it to the main entrance.

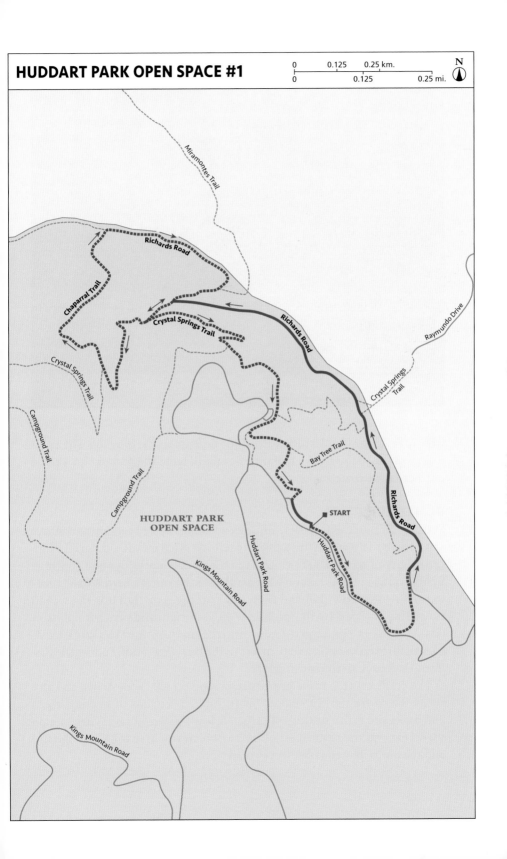

HUDDART PARK OPEN SPACE #1

0   0.125   0.25 km.

0   0.125   0.25 mi.

N

Miramontes Trail

Richards Road

Chaparral Trail

Crystal Springs Trail

Richards Road

Raymundo Drive

Crystal Springs Trail

Crystal Springs Trail

Campground Trail

Bay Tree Trail

Richards Road

HUDDART PARK
OPEN SPACE

START

Campground Trail

Huddart Park Road

Huddart Park Road

Kings Mountain Road

Kings Mountain Road

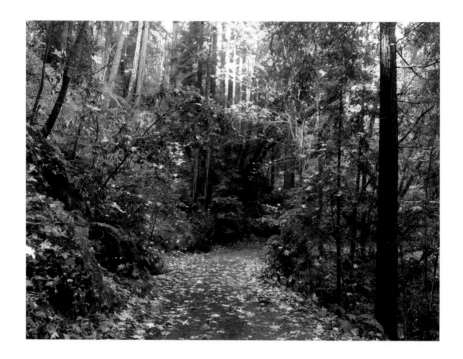

Continue down Huddart Park Road to the Sequoia parking lot. The trailhead is accessed less than a half mile downhill from the parking lot, on the left side of the road.

RUN DESCRIPTION

Starting on the doubletrack trail, descend amid forested canopy to connect with Richard's Road. After a quarter mile on Richard's Road, turn left up the spur trail to Crystal Springs Trail. Cross the footbridge and continue uphill and then turn right on Chaparral Trail. Rejoin Richard's Road, turning right to go downhill and then right on the spur trail (for the second time); this time pass by the footbridge on your right and turn left uphill on Crystal Springs Trail, about 2 miles into the run. Continue to a short, hard-packed dirt trail section and turn left to the Bay Tree Trail. Follow the Bay Tree Trail back to the parking lot.

The trails on this route are a mix of singletrack, wide trails, and fire roads. They are mostly smooth, with limited sections of exposed roots and rocks and many sections of carpeted, leaf-strewn terrain. There are no views beyond the ruggedness of the redwoods reaching high into the sky and the multicolored fallen leaves underfoot.

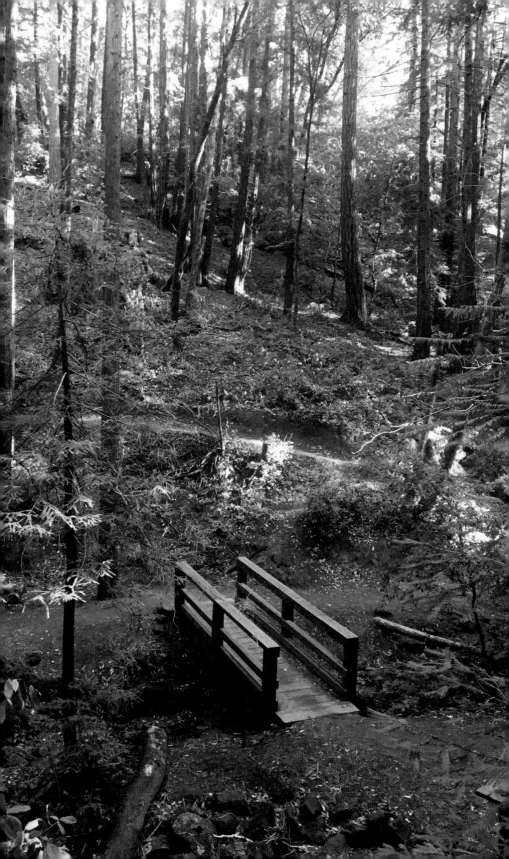

HUDDART PARK OPEN SPACE #2

THE RUNDOWN

START: Old Woodside Store; elevation 440 feet

OVERALL DISTANCE: 2.5-miles out and back with options for longer routes

APPROXIMATE RUNNING TIME: 25 minutes

DIFFICULTY: Green

ELEVATION GAIN: 182 feet

BEST SEASON TO RUN: Year-round

DOG FRIENDLY: No

PARKING: Free, but you must leave by 4 p.m., as gates will be locked.

OTHER USERS: Heavy equestrian, no bikes

CELL PHONE COVERAGE: Good

MORE INFORMATION: https://parks.smcgov.org/huddart-park

FINDING THE TRAILHEAD

Park at the Old Woodside Store at the intersection of Tripp Road and King's Mountain Road. The store, which doubles as a two-room museum complete with pioneer-style artifacts, is a San Mateo County Historic Site. There is a water spigot to top off water bottles. For this access to the park, a half-mile section along the road (there is a doubletrack dirt/gravel path parallel to the road) to the park entrance is required.

RUN DESCRIPTION

Start the run on King's Mountain Road, turning right on Greer Road. Turn left on Richards Road to enter the park. Numerous trail access points are available from this location. Return to the Woodside Store post-run for some rock candy.

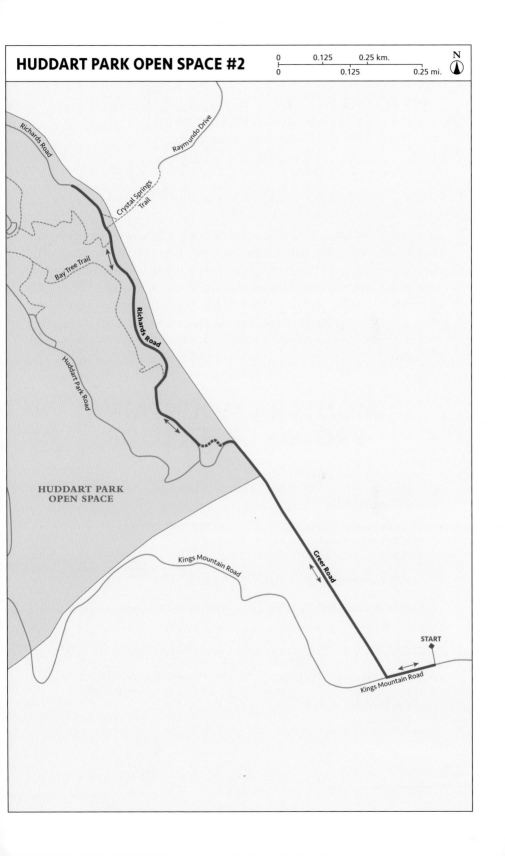

SAN PEDRO VALLEY REGIONAL PARK

LOCATED IN PACIFICA, THIS 1,052-ACRE PARK has a diverse network of more than 10 miles of singletrack, doubletrack, and gravel trail, complete with flat and ascending and descending sections. Although the trails are often within eucalyptus groves or hazelnut trees, there are also open views that, on a clear day, allow you to see Pacifica below and the Pacific Ocean to the west. The trails are well marked, and the two routes featured below offer very different experiences and, combined, make for a great 10 miles of trail running.

MONTARA MOUNTAIN/ BROOKS CREEK LOOP

THE RUNDOWN

START: Park entrance off Oddstad Boulevard; elevation 211 feet

OVERALL DISTANCE: 4.7 miles

APPROXIMATE RUNNING TIME: 60 minutes

DIFFICULTY: Blue

ELEVATION GAIN: 1,183 feet

BEST SEASON TO RUN: Year-round

DOG FRIENDLY: No

PARKING: Small fee, or purchase of an annual park pass

OTHER USERS: Cycling on paved trails

CELL PHONE COVERAGE: Good

MORE INFORMATION: https:// parks.smcgov.org/san-pedro -valley-park

MONTARA MOUNTAIN/BROOKS CREEK LOOP

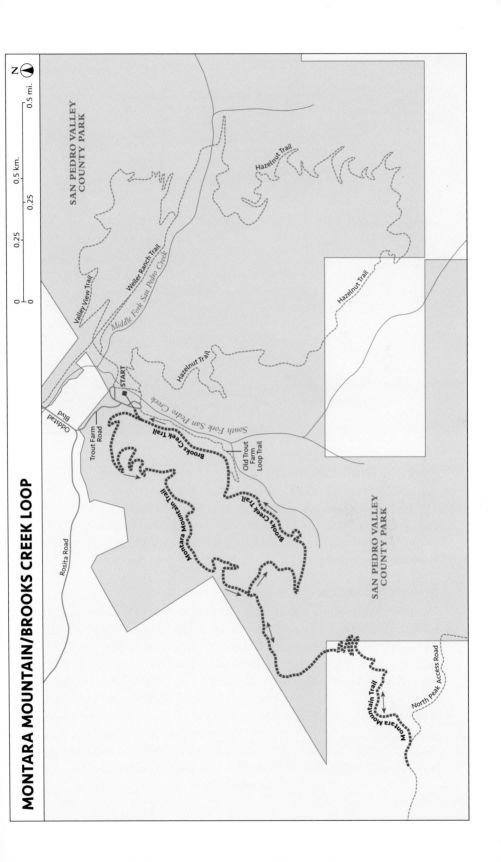

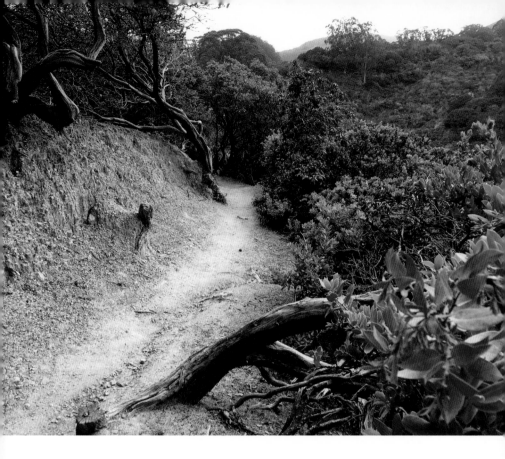

FINDING THE TRAILHEAD

Take the exit for CA 1 from I-280 and head south to the city of Pacifica. Turn east (left) onto Linda Mar Boulevard and follow it until it ends at Oddstad Boulevard, where you turn right and continue 1 block to the park entrance. The trailhead is located behind the restrooms across from the visitor center.

RUN DESCRIPTION

Turn right and follow the Montara Mountain Trail. On a clear day this smooth doubletrack trail affords views of the Pacific Ocean as well as glimpses of Montara Mountain. Much of the first three-quarters of a mile is shaded by towering eucalyptus trees and buffeted on either side of the trail by gnarly bushes and shrubs. Each quarter mile is signed. Approximately 1.75 miles into the run, turn right at the overlook sign to enjoy views of the ocean in the distance. One option is to make this a 3.5-mile out-and-back route. Continuing on past the overlook, cross the park boundary, where the trail becomes singletrack laden with rocks on long switchbacks with portions of wooden steps. At 2.4 miles into the run, reach Montara Road and make a choice to turn right on the dirt fire road to Montara Beach, turn left to Montara Mountain, or return on the trail from whence you came. If this is the option (as this route suggests), continue downhill to the junction of the Brooks Creek Trail on the right. This return provides a very different experience and makes a fantastic loop route. This mostly singletrack trail meanders through eucalyptus groves with pampas grasses shooting up from the hillside. Cross a footbridge and continue to a junction, taking the Old Trout Farm Trail to add distance to the run or following the Brooks Creek Trail back to the starting point for a 4.5-mile counterclockwise loop.

HAZELNUT TRAIL TO WEILER RANCH TRAIL LOOP

THE RUNDOWN

START: Park entrance off Oddstad Boulevard; elevation 179 feet

OVERALL DISTANCE: 4.8 miles

APPROXIMATE RUNNING TIME: 55 minutes

DIFFICULTY: Blue

ELEVATION GAIN: 861 feet

BEST SEASON TO RUN: Year-round

DOG FRIENDLY: No

PARKING: Small fee, or purchase of an annual park pass

OTHER USERS: Bikes on paved trails only

CELL PHONE COVERAGE: Good

MORE INFORMATION: https://parks.smcgov.org/locations/san-pedro-valley-park

FINDING THE TRAILHEAD

Take the exit for CA 1 from I-280 and head south to the city of Pacifica. Turn east (left) onto Linda Mar Boulevard and follow it until it ends at Oddstad Boulevard, where you turn right and continue 1 block to the park entrance. This trail starts to the right of the visitor center, crossing over a footbridge just beyond the interpretive signage.

RUN DESCRIPTION

After the footbridge turn right onto the Hazelnut Trail. Travel mostly uphill on a smooth, wide trail with many long switchbacks. Enjoy views of the Pacific Ocean to the west and wind through eucalyptus and hazelnut groves. After 1.75 miles of mostly uphill running, the remaining 2 miles of this trail is smooth singletrack, most of which is downhill. Every quarter mile is marked. Continue to the junction and turn left on a packed gravel path named the Weiler Ranch Trail. (If you turn right, you will reach the east end of the Weiler Ranch Trail, if you want to add mileage with an out-and-back route). Continue 0.4 mile over a footbridge. For additional mileage, turn right on the Valley View Trail for an extra 1.5-mile loop

HAZELNUT TRAIL TO WEILER RANCH TRAIL LOOP

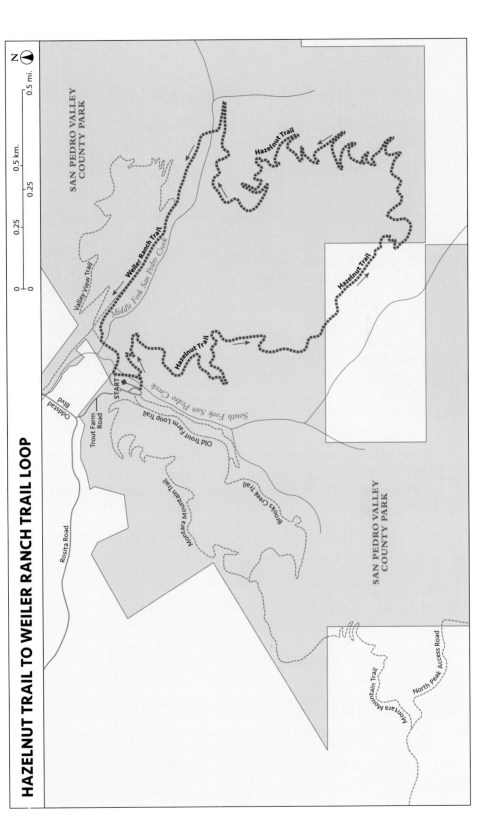

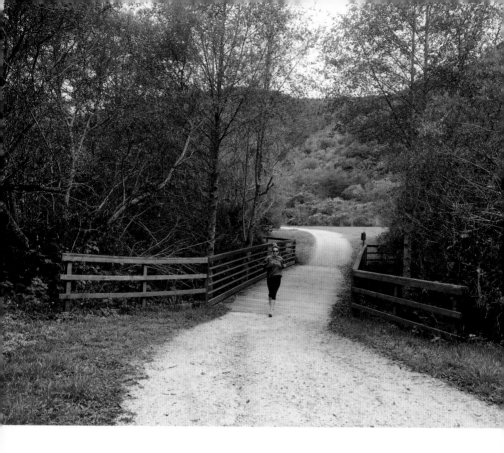

which rejoins Weiler Ranch Trail at its terminus, or, as this route suggests, continue to the parking lot, turning left on a short section of pavement to the Plaskon Nature Trail, which reaches the starting point at the Hazelnut Trail.

PACKS, HYDRATION SYSTEMS, GEL FLASKS, AND WATER FILTERS

Given the paucity of water fountains, spigots, or other conveniences on the typical trail run, most trail runners who run long enough to build up a thirst or hunger carry liquid and nutritional reserves. Depending on the temperature, projected length of run, availability of potable water, and particular hydration and nutritional needs of an individual trail runner, it may be necessary to carry substantial quantities of drink and food on a long trail excursion.

For shorter outings a trail runner is likely to be able to get by without any liquids or food. But as temperatures rise and the distance of a run lengthens, trail runners will, at a minimum, need to carry a 16- or 20-ounce bottle or flask of water or electrolyte-replacement sports drink. Depending on preference, bottles may be carried in hand, either by simply gripping the bottle or with the assistance of a strap that fastens the bottle around the back of the hand, or in a lumbar or "fanny" pack. Modern lumbar packs are designed to distribute weight evenly throughout the lumbar region and often feature straight or angled pouches for bottles and separate pockets for food, clothing, and accessories. Some lumbar packs also include "gel holsters" for runners who carry a gel flask. Gel flasks hold up to five packs of sports gel for easy consumption and relief from sticky fingers or the need to pack out trash.

For longer runs, especially on trails that do not come in contact with sources of potable water, a hydration pack or multibottle carrier is probably necessary. Hydration packs have become common accessories in the evolving world of endurance sports because of their convenience and functionality. They incorporate a bladder or reservoir, a delivery tube or hose, and a bite valve and allow trail runners to carry substantial quantities of fluid that are evenly distributed and consumed with hands-free ease. Other systems use a number of soft flasks that shrink when their contents are consumed. These are built more as form-fitting vests, with the flasks carried on the chest for easy access.

Hydration packs range in size and carrying capacity and come as backpacks, lumbar packs, and sports vests. Many hydration packs offer additional volume and storage pouches for food, clothing, and other trail necessities or conveniences. Certain bite valves are easier to use than others, and some bladders are difficult to clean or keep free of bacteria, mold, mildew, and fungus. Others come with antimicrobial compounds, and some feature in-line water filters.

When running on trails that cross water sources, whether streams, creeks, rivers, ponds, lakes, or merely large puddles, trail runners can free themselves of substantial weight by carrying water filters and a single water bottle. Make sure the filter removes such evils as *Cryptosporidium*, *Giardia*, *E. coli*, volatile organic compounds, and other threatening substances that are common to the area where it is likely to be used. Note, however, that water filters do not protect against viruses. It may be necessary to use a combination of iodine tablets with a filter to ensure the water is safe for consumption. Other devices use a charge to purify the water; another alternative is to use a filtered straw that allows you to pull filtered water directly from the source.

SKYLINE RIDGE OPEN SPACE PRESERVE

WITHIN THE MIDPENINSULA REGIONAL OPEN SPACE DISTRICT, there are 62,000 acres of preserved land within twenty-six open space preserves extending from San Carlos to Los Gatos and to the Pacific Ocean from south of Pacifica to the Santa Cruz County line. The Skyline Ridge Open Space Preserve offers 2,143 acres with more than 12 miles of trails. Wildflowers are abundant in the spring and summer, with some tree cover for shade, and open-space vistas. Beware of rattlesnakes on warm days. Trail markings are excellent.

IPIWA TRAIL LOOP

THE RUNDOWN

START: Preserve parking lot off Skyline Boulevard; elevation 2,085 feet

OVERALL DISTANCE: 2.6 miles

APPROXIMATE RUNNING TIME: 30 minutes

DIFFICULTY: Green

ELEVATION GAIN: 604 feet

BEST SEASON TO RUN: Year-round

DOG FRIENDLY: Leashed dogs on designated trails within the open space preserve but not on this particular route

PARKING: Free

OTHER USERS: Bicyclists, equestrians

CELL PHONE COVERAGE: Fair

MORE INFORMATION: www .openspace.org

IPIWA TRAIL LOOP

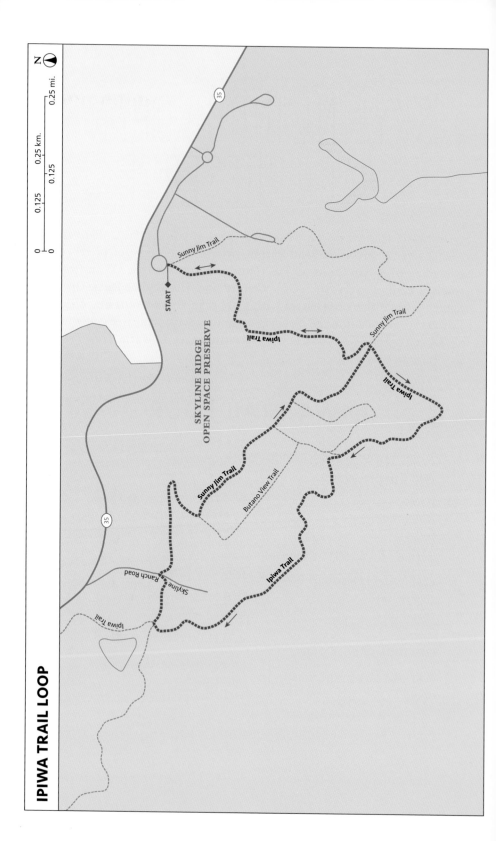

N

| 0 | 0.125 | 0.25 km. |
| 0 | 0.125 | 0.25 mi. |

35

Sunny Jim Trail

START

SKYLINE RIDGE
OPEN SPACE PRESERVE

Ipiwa Trail

Sunny Jim Trail

Ipiwa Trail

Sunny Jim Trail

Butano View Trail

35

Skyline Ranch Road

Ipiwa Trail

Ipiwa Trail

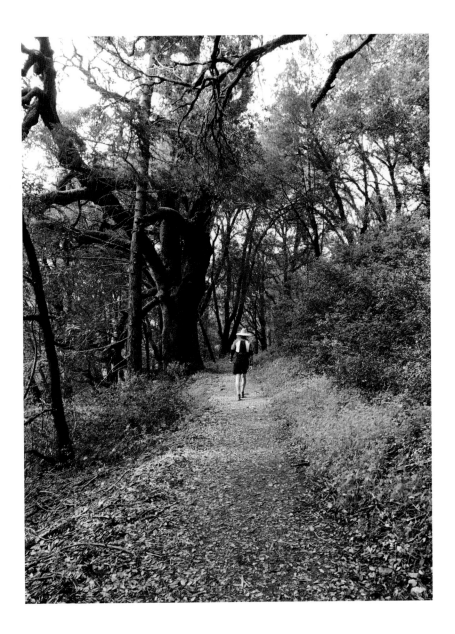

FINDING THE TRAILHEAD

Traveling north on Skyline Boulevard/CA 35 from CA 9, turn at the intersection on the south side of the road indicating the main preserve entrance, which is just before Page Mill Road. There is a restroom in the parking lot, and the trailhead is a tad beyond the interpretive signage on the southwest side of the parking lot.

RUN DESCRIPTION

Start uphill on the singletrack Ipiwa Trail, and immediately there are spectacular views before the trail enters a wooded section. Within a half mile the route reaches a clearing, and a connection to other signed trails. Continue straight along the Ipiwa Trail, winding to the west for more outstanding vistas that showcase the South Santa Cruz Mountains. Just beyond an overlook, return into the forest and turn right on the Sunny Jim Trail, which winds past park offices and a short, paved section. Follow signs to the right to continue on the Sunny Jim Trail, which connects back to the Ipiwa Trail, where you have the option of continuing straight for extra mileage to the Horseshoe Trail, which also leads back to the parking lot. For this route turn left on the Ipiwa Trail and return to the parking lot.

RUSSIAN RIDGE OPEN SPACE

CONNECTING TO THE SKYLINE RIDGE OPEN SPACE, the Russian Ridge section is 3,491 acres. In this location of abundant wildflowers, the green hills of winter and early spring turn to gold in summer. Featured views are of the San Francisco Bay and the Santa Cruz Mountains.

BOREL HILL OUT-AND-BACK

THE RUNDOWN

START: Russian Ridge parking lot off Alpine Road, La Honda; elevation 2,255 feet

OVERALL DISTANCE: 1.7 miles

APPROXIMATE RUNNING TIME: 20 minutes

DIFFICULTY: Green

ELEVATION GAIN: 292 feet

BEST SEASON TO RUN: Year-round

DOG FRIENDLY: Leashed dogs on designated trails within the open space preserve but not on this particular route

PARKING: Free

OTHER USERS: Bicyclists, equestrians

CELL PHONE COVERAGE: Fair

MORE INFORMATION: www .openspace.org

FINDING THE TRAILHEAD

 The parking lot is at the northwest corner of the intersection of Skyline Boulevard/CA 35 and Page Mill Road/Alpine Road.

BOREL HILL OUT-AND-BACK AT RUSSIAN RIDGE

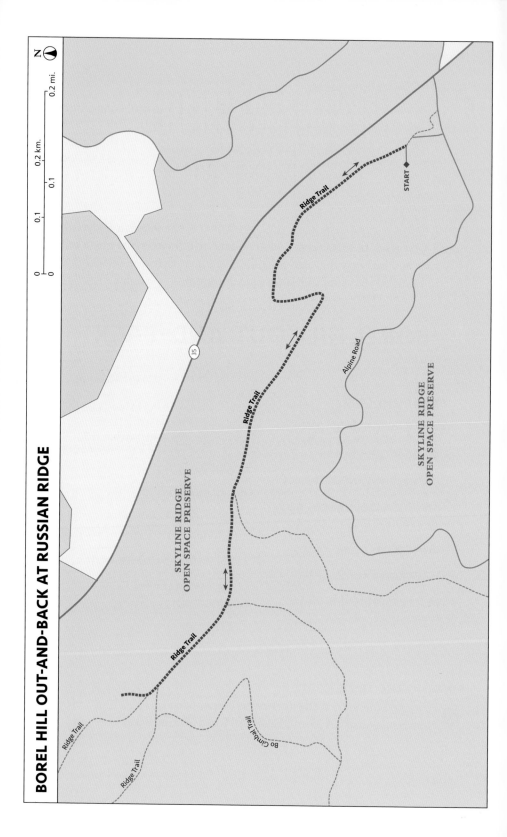

RUN DESCRIPTION

Enjoy this short out-and-back route that offers multiple trail connections for additional mileage. The trailhead is located on the northwest side of the parking lot. Start on doubletrack trail and continue on a gentle climb of doubletrack and singletrack trail to the Borel Hill viewpoint. This is the highest named peak in San Mateo County. Retrace your steps to return to the parking lot.

RANCHO CORRAL DE TIERRA

THE NEWEST ADDITION, in December 2011, to the Golden Gate National Recreation Area, Rancho Corral de Tierra covers 4,000 acres of open space. The trail system is not fully developed, and therefore the signage is not great. Carrying a map aids in having a positive experience on these trails, which are mostly in the open with views of the Pacific to the west and Montara Mountain to the north.

THE RUNDOWN

START: End of Coral Reef Avenue, Half Moon Bay; elevation 116 feet

OVERALL DISTANCE: 4 miles

APPROXIMATE RUNNING TIME: 45 minutes

DIFFICULTY: Blue

ELEVATION GAIN: 1,189 feet

BEST SEASON TO RUN: Year-round; beware of poison oak and muddy spots if rainy

DOG FRIENDLY: Dogs on leash

PARKING: Free

OTHER USERS: Cyclists and equestrians

CELL PHONE COVERAGE: Good

MORE INFORMATION: www.nps.gov/goga/rcdt.htm

FINDING THE TRAILHEAD

From CA 1, just south of the Half Moon Bay Airport, turn left on Coral Reef Avenue and follow the road to the end to park in this residential neighborhood on the cul-de-sac. The trailhead is on the north side of the parking area.

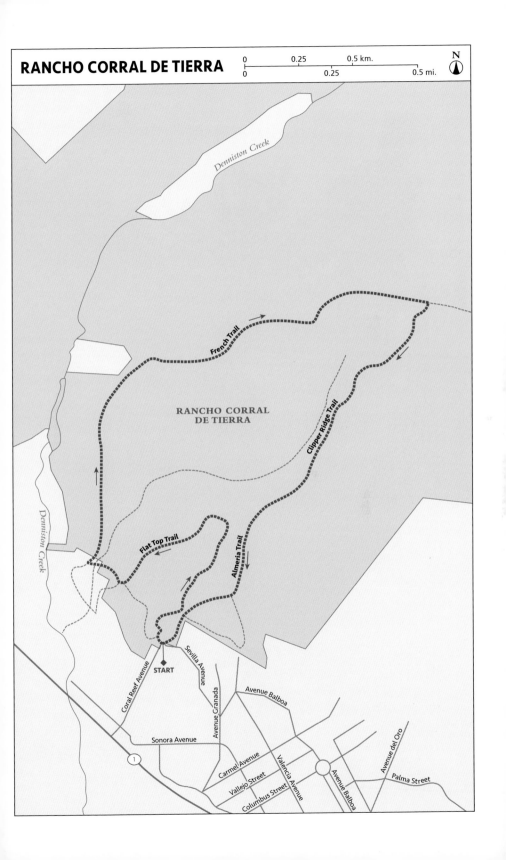

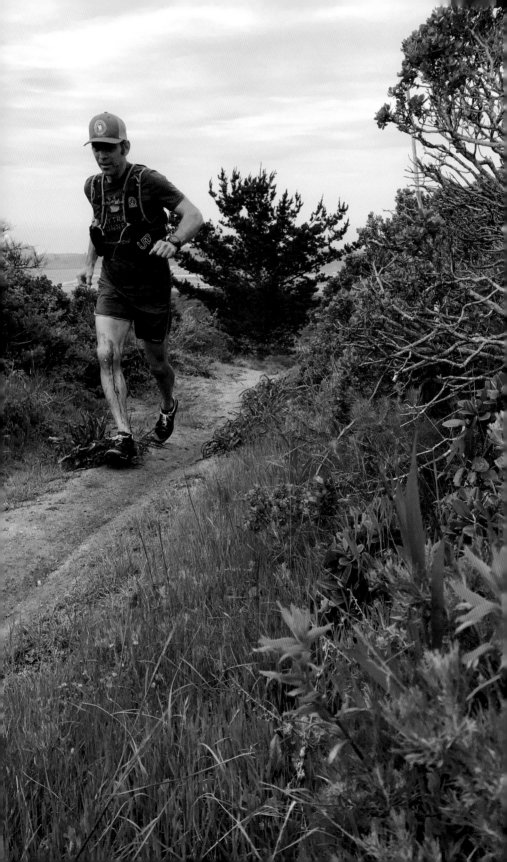

RUN DESCRIPTION

Start on a singletrack through pampas grasses, and pay attention not to go off-trail, where poison oak encounters are common. After a half mile of mostly ascending, turn left down a steep hill and then turn right at the bottom, which leads to a creek crossing and a boggy section. Climb for nearly 1.5 miles and turn right at the intersection; then descend for much of the way back to the parking area. This route offers amazing views throughout and provides a challenge with climbing and descending. The variety of wildflowers adds to the allure of what is currently a low-use area.

PENINSULA

RUNNING GEAR

EYEWEAR

Running eyewear has progressed enormously in the last decade, to the point that sunglasses are now functional and extremely protective (as well as looking pretty cool). Because trail runners constantly use their eyes to scope out their next steps and enjoy the awesome views, the eyes are very valuable assets—and worth preserving. With lighter frames, full protection from harmful ultraviolet rays, and lenses that shield eyes from insects, dirt, and shrubbery, modern glasses are worth wearing.

Today's eyewear also tends to be versatile, sporting features such as adjustable bridges and temples and interchangeable lenses to accommodate changes in brightness. Some sports glasses have venting features that prevent lenses from fogging. Other attributes to consider include rubberized bridges to prevent slipping and straight or wraparound frames that relieve temple pressure. Photochromic lenses are particularly well suited for trails because they adjust to the lighting, getting darker when exposed to more sun and lighter (and even clear) when in the shade or dark.

When shopping for trail-running eyewear, look for lenses that offer full UV protection. Sports eyewear prices range dramatically. Make sure the glasses have the features that are most desirable—lightweight, fit, UV protection, and high resolution—before buying a pair of cheap gas station glasses or investing a week's wages in some designer shades.

ELECTRONICS

Although trail runners are better known for their back-to-nature approach and avoiding modern technological devices—especially when compared to road runners, mountain bikers, or triathletes (aka "tri-geeks")—certain gadgets add to the trail-running experience and can be used discreetly or, in some cases, rather boldly, as when shared on social media. A cell phone carried in a hydration pack can be a lifesaver in the event of an emergency, as is the case with a satellite phone or tracker device.

Watches have come a long way since the days of just telling the time of day and perhaps the date. Now they are "wrist-top computers" or "action trackers" capable of telling distance traveled, speed, leg speed cadence, direction, barometric pressure, weather trends, altitude, heart rate, and ascent and descent rates; and they can even receive and transmit messages. Whether knowing any of that data is desirable is a subjective question, but some of it can be quite motivational, assist coaches, and make us safer. Trail runners are now able to explore new terrain with fewer worries of getting hopelessly lost or being hit by an unexpected storm. Neither will we have an excuse for being late.

Flashlights and headlamps are important devices for trail runners who run in the dark, especially ultradistance runners, who are likely to race or train at night. Many types of flashlights and headlamps are on the market, so weigh anticipated needs against the different attributes of various light sources. A flashlight provides precise directional focus but usually requires one hand to hold it. In contrast, headlamps free the hands, but some runners find that the light angle makes it difficult to discern trail obstacles because it shines from above.

Flashlights and headlamps come in different weights and brightnesses and with a variety of light sources, such as halogen, fluorescent, LED (light-emitting diodes), and conventional and somewhat outdated tungsten bulb lights. These different types of light vary in brightness, energy efficiency, durability, and cost. Some units allow for adjustability in brightness and intensity of focus, while others come with rechargeable battery packs and water-resistant or waterproof qualities.

MISCELLANEOUS GEAR

Thanks to the influence of Nordic skiers, adventure racers, and European trail runners, the use of lightweight trekking poles has increased. Runners use these collapsible poles to help redistribute the workload from the legs to the upper body, especially on ascents. Poles also help with balance. They should be light, sturdy, and easy to carry when not in use. If the poles have baskets, they should be minimal in size in order to avoid entanglements and reduce awkwardness in use. While sharp points make the poles excellent spears for charging beasts, they can also do a fine job on one's own feet.

Trail runners should also consider wearing low-cut gaiters, even when there is no snow around. Gaiters prevent gravel, scree, sand, stones, and dirt from penetrating the ankle collar of shoes, thus relieving trail runners from the frustration of running with a buildup of trail debris at the bottom of their shoes or the annoyance of having to stop to remove the offend-ing substance from shoe and sock. Some trail shoes are now designed with gaiter attachments or snug-fitting ankle collars to prevent any intrusion of debris.

From the safety perspective, trail runners may consider carrying a first-aid kit, snakebite kit, or basic backcountry safety items like a lighter, about 20 feet of lightweight rope, and a Swiss Army knife, Leatherman, or other multipurpose tool. Maps are also very useful. It might also be wise to pack a whistle or mace to repel uninvited advances, whether animal or human. Consider bringing duct tape—the universal solution, panacea, and fix-all that works in a pinch as a makeshift gaiter, blister preventer or mender, cut patcher, splint, tourniquet, garment rip stopper, etc. In sum, if a trail emergency can't be remedied with duct tape, it's time for grave concern.

Devoted trail runners may need some added traction before braving our icy winter and spring trails. Footwear traction devices come in sev-eral varieties, and depending on the extensiveness of ice, depth of snow, and prevalence of rocks and other hard surfaces under and surrounding the ice, trail runners will want to select the appropriate aggressiveness and materials of the device's teeth. Some traction devices have relatively shal-low teeth that are made with softer substances, like rubber or plastic, while others feature long, fang-like claws made of metal alloys. Other options are to attach Icespikes or use wood screws which can be drilled directly into the outsole of your shoes. As well, you can purchase special winterized trail shoes that feature carbide tips.

For those who run with canine companions, some of the leashes on the market make life a lot easier. There are "hands-free" leashes that are worn around the waist and attach to the dog's collar via quick-release mecha-nisms for safety and convenience. Other leashes are made from elastic shock cord to allow some play without excessive slack, a real convenience when trails are rocky or otherwise require quick maneuvers that may not coincide with the movements of the dog.

Another handy item is a leash pack, which conveniently slides over a leash to carry "poop bags," both empty and full. Collapsible lightweight bowls that pack onto a leash or into a fanny pack make it easy to keep four-legged trail runners well hydrated and fed on the run.

QUARRY PARK

IN THE SAN MATEO COUNTY PARK SYSTEM, the 517-acre Quarry Park may be small, but the trail system connects to that of Rancho to the northwest and Miranda Surf to the south, reaching the Coastal Trail in less than 1.5 miles.

THE RUNDOWN

START: Santa Maria Avenue, Half Moon Bay; elevation 126 feet

OVERALL DISTANCE: 2 miles

APPROXIMATE RUNNING TIME: 22 minutes

DIFFICULTY: Green, but some decent climbing

ELEVATION GAIN: 500 feet

BEST SEASON TO RUN: Year-round; avoid in heavy rain or wind.

DOG FRIENDLY: Dogs on leash

PARKING: Free

OTHER USERS: Equestrians, bicyclists on service roads only

CELL PHONE COVERAGE: Good

MORE INFORMATION: https:// parks.smcgov.org/quarry-park

PENINSULA

FINDING THE TRAILHEAD

From CA 1 in Half Moon Bay, head east on Capistrano Road, turn right on Alhambra Avenue, then left on Avenue Cabrillo, left on Columbus Street, and right on Santa Maria Avenue. Parking is on the left, and the trailhead is just beyond the gate, across from the playground and restroom.

RUN DESCRIPTION

Start in an open meadow, and within a few hundred feet this wide dirt and gravel path ascends on a gentle climb through eucalyptus groves for about three-quarters of a mile. Numerous leaves blanket the ground, as well as downed tree branches and eucalyptus bark, so watch your footing. Turn right at the next two intersections, and feel free to stop to enjoy a glimpse

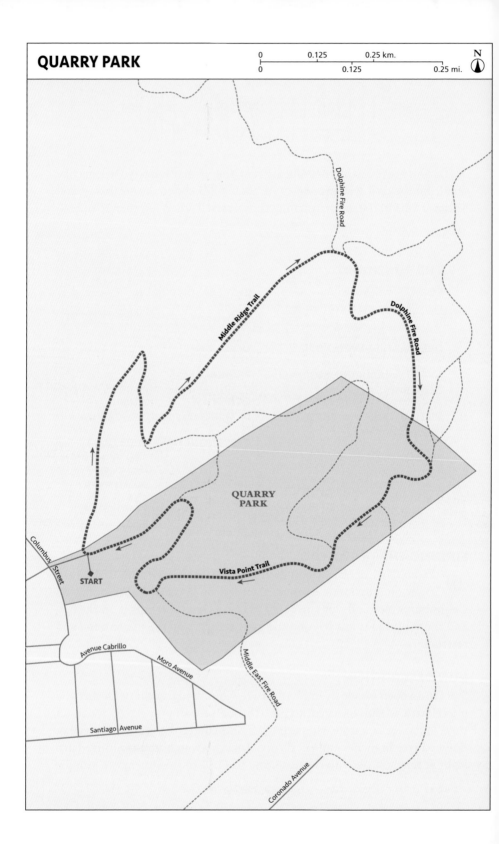

QUARRY PARK

0   0.125   0.25 km.
0   0.125   0.25 mi.

N

Dolphine Fire Road

Middle Ridge Trail

Dolphine Fire Road

QUARRY
PARK

Vista Point Trail

Columbus Street

START

Avenue Cabrillo

Moro Avenue

Middle East Fire Road

Santiago Avenue

Coronado Avenue

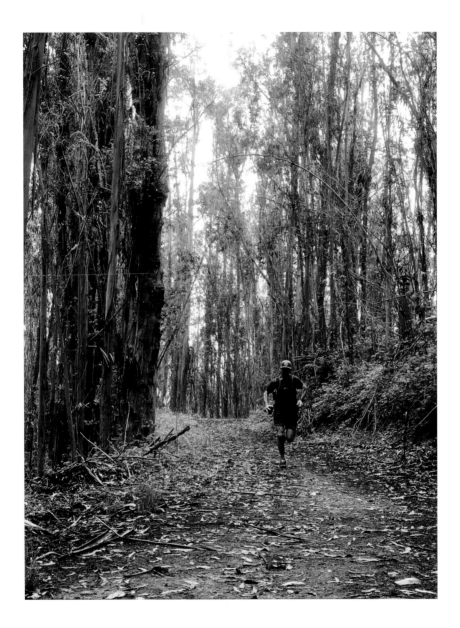

of the ocean at a well-placed park bench. Descend on the trail back to the parking lot. The majority of the route is within the forest. Even though there are only 4 miles of trails, be sure to carry a map, as the trails are not well signed.

EDGEWOOD PARK AND NATURAL PRESERVE

THIS 467-ACRE PARK in the San Mateo County Park system offers 10 miles of extremely well-signed trails. The mostly singletrack rolling trails are complete with long switchbacks, both climbing and descending in the forest and through open meadows.

THE RUNDOWN

START: Edgewood Park parking area; elevation 245 feet

OVERALL DISTANCE: 3.8 miles

APPROXIMATE RUNNING TIME: 40 minutes

DIFFICULTY: Green

ELEVATION GAIN: 677 feet

BEST SEASON TO RUN: Year-round

DOG FRIENDLY: No

PARKING: Free on street; small day-use fee to park in main lot, or purchase of an annual park pass

OTHER USERS: Most trails are open to equestrians; no bikes.

CELL PHONE COVERAGE: Poor, unless AT&T (then it is marginal)

MORE INFORMATION: https://parks.smcgov.org/edgewood-park-trails

FINDING THE TRAILHEAD

From I-280 take the Edgewood Road exit. Head east on Edgewood Road (toward San Carlos and Redwood City) for approximately 1.5 miles. The main park entrance is on the south side of the road. There is some off-street parking along Edgewood Road just outside the park entrance. Cross over the boardwalk to the trailhead. Check out details on the free weekend park shuttle, as the area is crowded on the weekends.

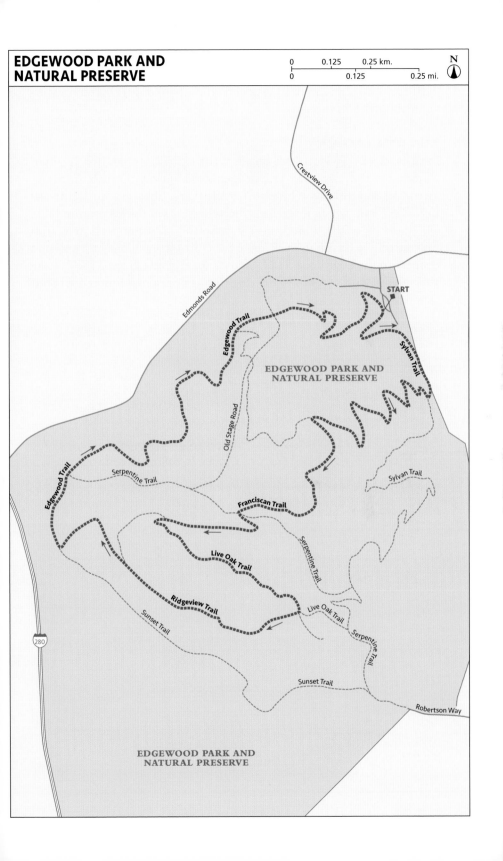

EDGEWOOD PARK AND
NATURAL PRESERVE

0   0.125   0.25 km.

0   0.125   0.25 mi.

N

Crestview Drive

Edmonds Road

Edgewood Trail

START

Sylvan Trail

EDGEWOOD PARK AND
NATURAL PRESERVE

Old Stage Road

Edgewood Trail

Serpentine Trail

Sylvan Trail

Franciscan Trail

Live Oak Trail

Serpentine Trail

Ridgeview Trail

Sunset Trail

Live Oak Trail

280

Serpentine Trail

Sunset Trail

Robertson Way

EDGEWOOD PARK AND
NATURAL PRESERVE

There are two alternative access points for off-street parking along with the main park entrance lot.

RUN DESCRIPTION

For this clockwise loop start on the Sylvan Trail. At the first junction continue on the Franciscan Trail, which winds mostly through the forest, ascending on gentle switchbacks. Turn left after about 1.5 miles onto the Live Oak Trail, which is reached after crossing over the Serpentine Trail. The majority of the climb is nearly complete. At just under 2 miles, follow the trail to the right, the Ridgeview Trail, for about one half-mile and connect to the Edgewood Trail. Enjoy a long, gentle descent back to the parking lot, with sections wandering through open meadow and wooded canopy.

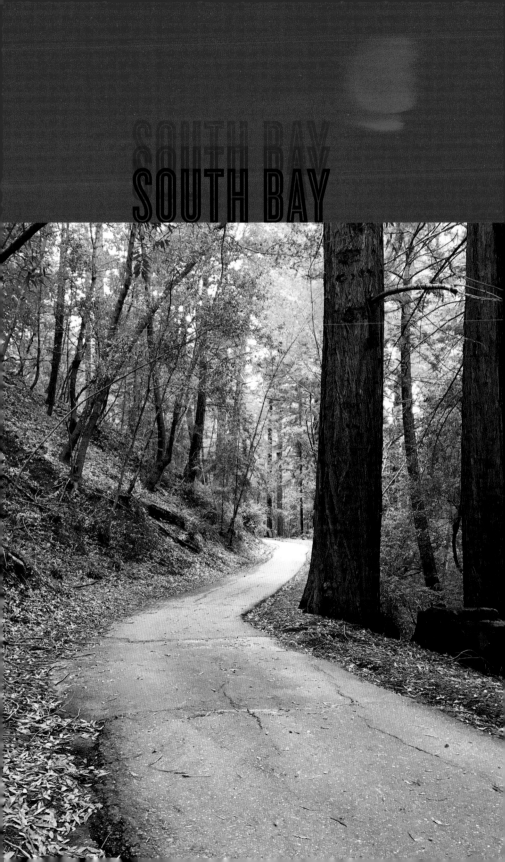

SIERRE AZUL OPEN SPACE PRESERVE/ ALMADEN QUICKSILVER COUNTY PARK

TRANSLATED AS "BLUE RANGE," the Sierre Azul Open Space covers more than 18,000 acres and provides numerous opportunities for loop, out-and-back, or point-to-point routes. Trails are primarily fire roads and double-track, but with the opening of the Mount Umunhum Trail in September 2017, a 4.5-mile round-trip on singletrack is accessible, starting at the top of the paved road leading to Mount Umunhum. Offering shaded sections featuring California bay laurel, as well as open areas with expansive views of the Santa Clara Valley (and from Mount Umunhum, 360-degree views from this 3,486-foot summit), this rural area is not far from the suburbs. Almaden Quicksilver County Park encompasses 4,163 acres, including Capitancillos Ridge. With three access points to trailheads, more than 37 miles of trails await, offering a mix of singletrack and fire roads. Bikers and equestrians are permitted, as are leashed dogs.

SIERRE AZUL OPEN SPACE PRESERVE/ALMADEN QUICKSILVER COUNTY PARK

THE RUNDOWN

START: Woods Trail parking lot off Hicks Road; elevation 1,416 feet

OVERALL DISTANCE: 3.1 miles

APPROXIMATE RUNNING TIME: 30 minutes

DIFFICULTY: Green

ELEVATION GAIN: 335 feet

BEST SEASON TO RUN: Year-round

DOG FRIENDLY: Leashed dogs on designated trails

PARKING: Free

OTHER USERS: Equestrians and mountain bikes on designated trails

CELL PHONE COVERAGE: Fair to marginal

MORE INFORMATION: www .openspace.org/preserves/ sierra-azul; www.sccgov.org/ sites/parks/parkfinder/Pages/ AlmadenPark.aspx

SOUTH BAY

FINDING THE TRAILHEAD

There are several access points to the park. This route starts at the Hicks Road entrance. Follow CA 85 to the Camden Avenue exit in San Jose. Take Camden Avenue south and turn right on Hicks Road. Follow Hicks Road to the parking lot at the Woods Trail trailhead near the intersection of Mount Umunhum Road. Across Hicks Road is one of the many trailheads for Almaden Quicksilver. There is a toilet at this staging area.

RUN DESCRIPTION

Start just beyond the gate and follow the Woods Trail for this out-and-back route. The route winds in and out of shade on a wide, mostly smooth trail. There are limited views on this route, but as you ascend and continue

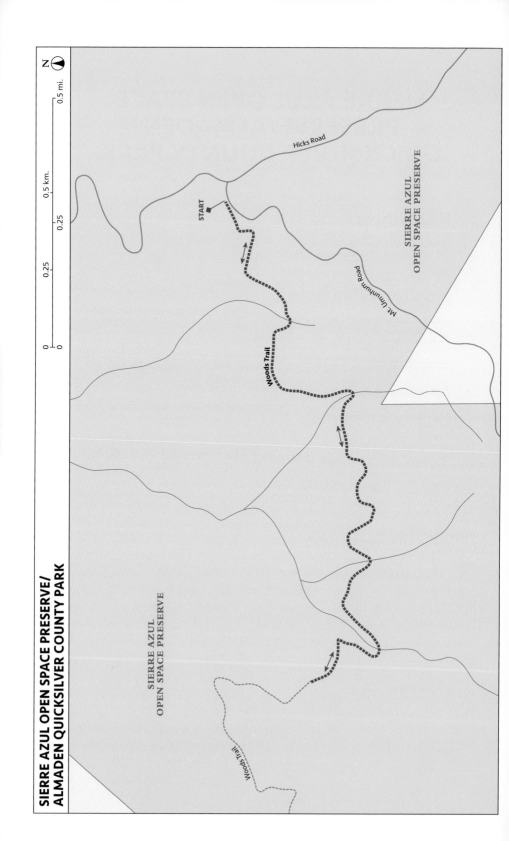

SIERRE AZUL OPEN SPACE PRESERVE/
ALMADEN QUICKSILVER COUNTY PARK

N

0.5 mi.

0.5 km.

0.25

0.25

0

0

Hicks Road

START

Mt. Umunhum Road

Woods Trail

SIERRE AZUL
OPEN SPACE PRESERVE

SIERRE AZUL
OPEN SPACE PRESERVE

Woods Trail

up the Woods Trail, there are great views. Starting on the Woods Trail, you can create a 7-mile loop that includes the Barlow Road (a fire road) and Mount Umunhum Road (paved) for a return to the starting point (see route below).

WOODS TRAIL LOOP

FINDING THE TRAILHEAD

There are several access points to the park. This route starts at the Hicks Road entrance. Follow CA 85 to the Camden Avenue exit in San Jose. Take Camden Avenue south and turn right on Hicks Road. Follow Hicks Road to the parking lot at the Woods Trail trailhead near the intersection of Mount Umunhum Road. Across Hicks Road is one of the many trailheads for Almaden Quicksilver. There is a toilet at this staging area.

RUN DESCRIPTION

Run on the Woods Trail, a relatively smooth-surfaced trail with a gentle climb. After about 2.8 miles, turn left on Barlow Road and follow for approximately 2 miles most of which is uphill with some of the steepest climbing (some upwards of 15 percent grade) in the first half mile. There is a slight downhill section and a short saddle and then another climb that reaches the highest point on this route at just over 2,400 feet at the 4.7-mile point and the junction of Mount Umunhum Road. Turn left on Mount Umunhum Road to return to the starting point, descending all the way.

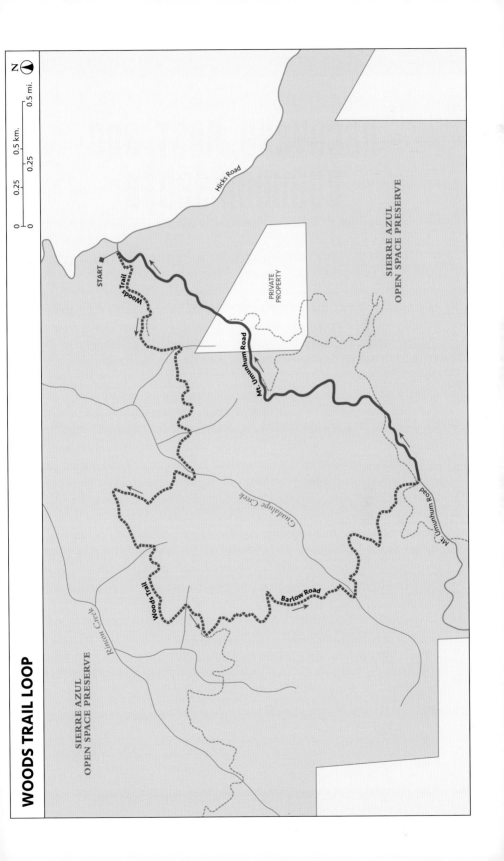

WOODS TRAIL LOOP

N

0   0.25   0.5 km.
0   0.25   0.5 mi.

Hicks Road

START

Woods Trail

Mt. Umunhum Road

PRIVATE PROPERTY

SIERRE AZUL OPEN SPACE PRESERVE

Guadalupe Creek

Woods Trail

Rincon Creek

SIERRE AZUL OPEN SPACE PRESERVE

Barlow Road

Mt. Umunhum Road

RECOVERY, REST, and COMMON SENSE

More is not always better. This is sometimes the most difficult lesson for trail runners to fully absorb. Failure to learn the lesson leads to acute injury or chronic suboptimal performance. Even ultrarunners know that some rest, even if only active rest through cross-training, enhances their running performance. Just as the need exists to integrate recovery and rest into repeat or interval training to get the most from each repeat or interval, periods of recovery and rest should be integrated into your overall training schedule. It often takes more discipline to take a day off than to go hard or long.

With proper recovery and rest, trail runners are able to attack hard days and make them worthwhile. Without recovery and rest, the pace of hard runs and easy runs will be approximately the same, and very little benefit will result from either. If you are the type who is likely to overdo it, keep a running log or journal that tracks your daily runs, noting time, effort, mileage, and other pertinent factors such as weather, cross-training activities, sleep, diet, workload, emotional state, stress level, terrain, and, if you know them, altitude and heart rate. Those daily entries will force you to face the question of whether you are doing quality runs as opposed to sheer quantity. The diary will also give an indication of whether you are overtraining. When you notice progress in your running, you will be in a better position to recall and evaluate what factors worked to produce that success.

Another alternative for those who lack the discipline for proper recovery and rest is to get a coach. Although not many coaches specialize in trail training, a good running coach will be able to help develop a customized training schedule that takes into consideration a runner's personal strengths and weaknesses. A coach should also help integrate recovery days and rest into your training.

Only so much fuel is in any runner's tank, and if it isn't replenished between workouts, that reservoir will soon be running on empty. While it is a worthwhile training experience to overstress your system and run on "fumes," that should be a rare exception rather than the rule. Depriving the body of proper recovery and rest is like running without adequate food or drink; eventually breakdown will occur, at which point you'll have to stop for longer than you would had you worked adequate recovery and rest periods into the training schedule.

To ensure that easy days or recovery runs are not overly strenuous, arrange to run with someone who is willing to run at a moderate pace. Avoid running with someone who has a proclivity to pick it up or with whom you tend to be competitive. Consider running without a watch, or wear a heart rate monitor that can be set to warn if a predetermined rate is exceeded. Be open to the idea of walking ascents, stopping to stretch, or simply smelling the flowers and enjoying a vista.

A trail runner may boast of having put in a solid month of 120-mile weeks yet show little to no benefit from such high mileage. Alternatively, a runner who puts in as little as 30 to 40 miles a week in three or four runs can show tremendous progress if each of those runs serves a particular training purpose. Design the easy days to accomplish a purpose, and transfer any pent-up energy to the hard or long days to really make those workouts count toward improvement.

Although trail running may not beat a runner up the way road or track running does, it is still important to incorporate recovery and rest into training. Recovery and rest periods should come between repeats and intervals, between hard workouts, and before and after races. The use of recovery and rest also applies on a macro level, such as in scheduling a particular season or year to build up to a specific running goal. A trail runner often picks a race as far off as a year, then trains with that race in mind, perhaps running several "training" races geared to preparing for "the target" race.

The training principle of "periodization" (also called "phase" training) is based on the idea that an athlete may reach a performance peak by building up through a set of steps, each of which may last for weeks or months, depending on the starting point and where the athlete wants to be at the peak of the periodization training. Periodization training starts with a buildup or foundation period, upon which is built a base of endurance and strength. From there, the athlete works on speed and endurance, incorporating distance, tempo runs, intervals, repeats, and fartleks. Once the fitness and strength levels are sufficient to run the target distance at a pace that is close to the goal, focus is reoriented to speed work and turnover to tweak muscles for a fast pace. It is at this point that the athlete is ready for a recovery phase, also known as the "taper" period.

Within the big picture of a periodization schedule, you should be prepared to make micro adjustments for recovery and rest to stave off overtraining or injury. Know your body and be aware of heightened heart rate; sleep problems; loss of appetite; tight or sore muscles, bones, and connective tissue; a short temper; a general lack of enthusiasm; or other symptoms of burnout. Get adequate sleep with a consistent sleep routine. Quality of rest is probably more important than quantity, and playing catch-up does not always work to restore your body to a rested state. Also be sure to eat a balanced diet with adequate calories and fluids to power through the workout and the entire day.

Engaging in yoga or meditation can play a useful part in the recovery and rest phase. Just because you are not running trails during your time off doesn't mean you must sacrifice the peace of mind gained from running in a beautiful place. Those who practice meditative arts are able to reach a similar state of equanimity and tranquility to that gained by running trails, without lifting a foot. Another restorative measure, if available, is a sauna, hot tub, or steam room. The benefits of sports massage are also likely to be worth the time and cost.

When determining the amount of recovery and rest needed, consider the impact of other life events and the effect that family, work, travel, social, and emotional lives have on training—and vice versa. The need may arise to run more or less during particularly stressful periods, regardless of the specific point in the periodization schedule. If you are emotionally drained, a long, slow run in a scenic environment might replace what was supposed to be a hard hill repeat day.

Know yourself, set reasonable short- and long-term goals, and be willing to adjust them. Be flexible and avoid imposing on yourself a training partner's or someone else's goals. Every trail runner is an individual and responds to different types of training. What works for one trail runner might be a huge mistake for another. Be sensitive to all of your needs, plus those of family, friends, and coworkers.

A holistic approach to trail running will keep training in perspective. Yes, you need to respect the importance of adequate training, but do not miss the forest for the trees. You will be better able to run the trail that leads through those trees if you do it from a more balanced place. In addition to proper form, fitness, strength, nutrition, and gear, athletes become better runners if they are happy with their family and work lives. Avoiding overtraining or chronic fatigue and approaching each run with fervor keeps a runner motivated and ensures quality training. You will also run more easily if not burdened with stress or lack of recovery, rest, and relaxation. Finally, common sense trumps total exhaustion, lasting pain, and serious injury.

Running trails with a sense of purpose and strength is an invigorating experience that cultivates a deep sensation of satisfaction, one that overflows and leads to a fulfilling life.

SANBORN COUNTY PARK

NESTLED AMID LUSH FOREST, this 3,453-acre park is located just a few minutes' drive from the town of Saratoga, where, following a run, one can enjoy expensive treats while shopping or a Michelin-rated dinner at the Plumed Horse. This Santa Clara County park boasts 22 miles of trails with a mix of singletrack and doubletrack, smooth and technical terrain. The San Andreas Fault runs through the middle of the park. Because there is picnicking and camping, the area can become crowded during late spring and summer, especially on weekends. Even when busy, this park is an enjoyable escape in the woods from the heat of summer.

SANBORN COUNTY PARK #1

THE RUNDOWN

START: Parking lot off Sanborn Road; elevation 1,380 feet

OVERALL DISTANCE: 3 miles

APPROXIMATE RUNNING TIME: 35 minutes

DIFFICULTY: Blue

ELEVATION GAIN: 662 feet

BEST SEASON TO RUN: Year-round

DOG FRIENDLY: Leashed pets in designated areas

PARKING: Day-use fee

OTHER USERS: Bicyclists on designated trails; no equestrians

CELL PHONE COVERAGE: Poor

MORE INFORMATION: www .sccgov.org/sites/parks/ parkfinder/pages/sanborn .aspx

SANBORN COUNTY PARK #1

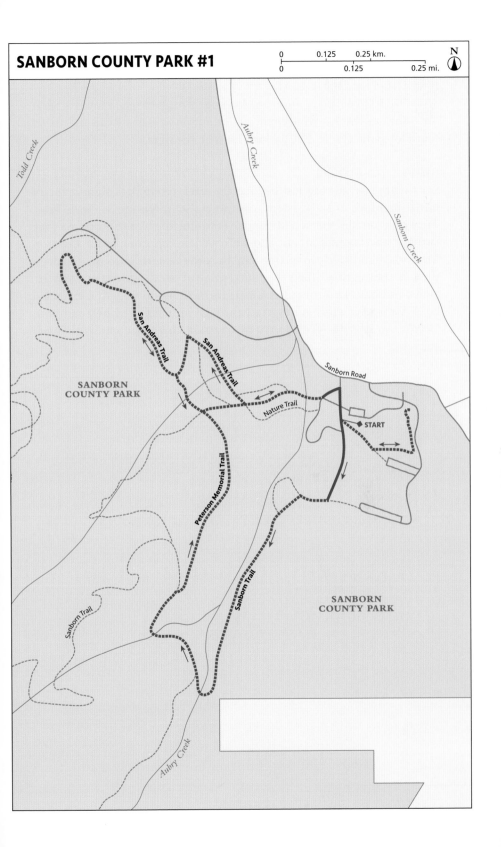

0   0.125   0.25 km.

0   0.125   0.25 mi.

N

Todd Creek

Aubry Creek

Sanborn Creek

San Andreas Trail

San Andreas Trail

Sanborn Road

Nature Trail

SANBORN
COUNTY PARK

START

Peterson Memorial Trail

Sanborn Trail

Sanborn Trail

SANBORN
COUNTY PARK

Aubry Creek

FINDING THE TRAILHEAD

From CA 85 follow Saratoga Avenue through the glam town of Saratoga to CA 9, a windy road. Turn left on Sanborn Road and travel south for about a mile. The parking lot is on the right.

RUN DESCRIPTION

Start on the paved road just beyond the interpretive park signage for an initial half mile of steep ascent, continuing south on the Sanborn Trail. Turn right on the Peterson Memorial Trail and follow it to portions of the San Andreas Trail for an out-and-back section, returning to the Peterson Memorial Trail for a connecting loop back to the starting point. Although there is trail signage along the route, some of the directional arrows are a bit confusing. This route has a mixture of technical singletrack; several creek crossings; wide, grassy trail through an open meadow; and both ascents and descents. With a variety of terrain, this park appeals to a broad audience.

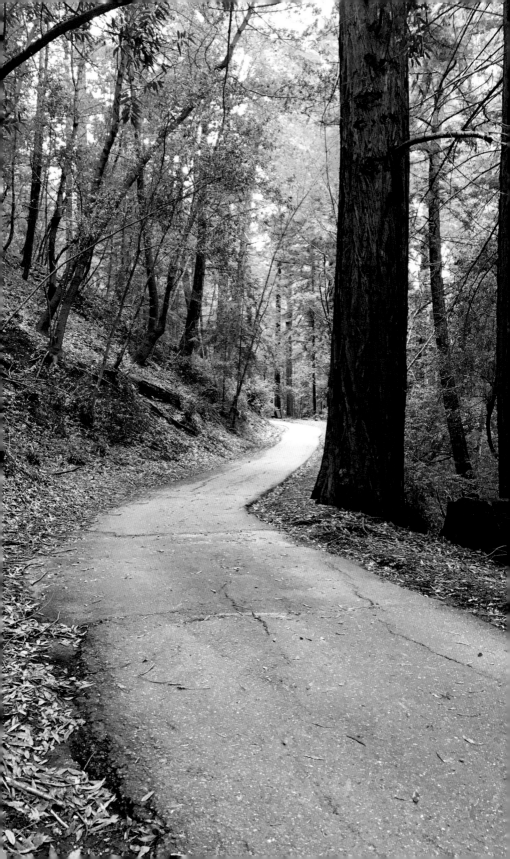

SANBORN COUNTY PARK #2

THE RUNDOWN

START: Parking lot off Sanborn Road; elevation 1,380 feet

OVERALL DISTANCE: 11 miles

APPROXIMATE RUNNING TIME: 105 minutes

DIFFICULTY: Blue

ELEVATION GAIN: 2,661 feet

BEST SEASON TO RUN: Year-round

DOG FRIENDLY: Leashed pets in designated areas

PARKING: Day-use fee

OTHER USERS: Bicyclists on designated trails; no equestrians

CELL PHONE COVERAGE: Marginal

MORE INFORMATION: www .sccgov.org/sites/parks/ parkfinder/pages/sanborn .aspx

FINDING THE TRAILHEAD

From CA 85 follow Saratoga Avenue through the glam town of Saratoga to CA 9, a windy road. Turn left on Sanborn Road and travel south for about a mile. The parking lot is on the right.

RUN DESCRIPTION

For a longer journey start on the Sanborn Trail and turn south (left) to meet up with the Skyline Trail, a mostly singletrack trail, and head west. There is also the option to head east to meet up with the switchbacks of the John Nicholas Trail. For this route, however, continue past Indian Rock and Summit Rock, or turn back to shorten the run. The Skyline Trail will reach the adjoining Castle Rock State Park to the northwest. There are two short out-and-backs on this route near the Summit Rock area, just to give a look at the cool rocks. There is also a spot here where you could end if someone picked you up.

SANBORN COUNTY PARK #2

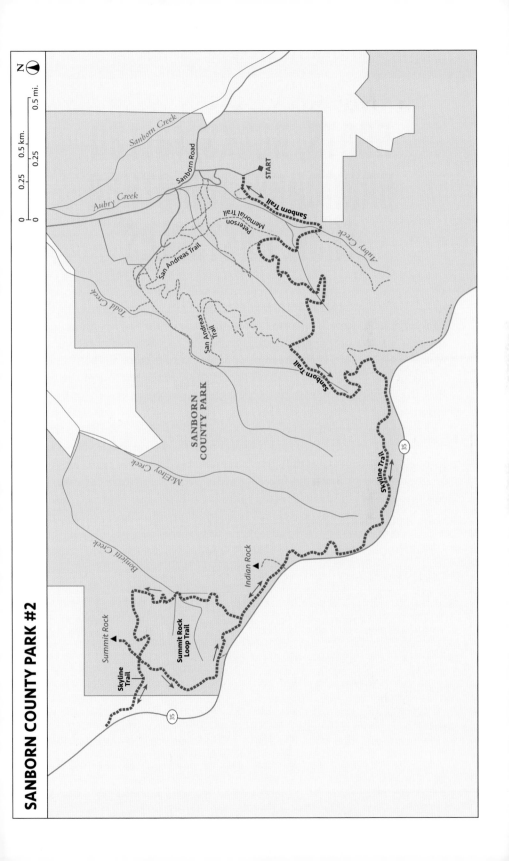

ROOTS, ROCKS, FALLEN BRANCHES, AND OTHER TRAIL OBSTACLES

When running on a particularly difficult section of trail, it is often beneficial to lift your knees a little higher than usual. This will give your feet more ground clearance to avoid catching a toe or otherwise tripping on a rock, root, or other potential snag. Using the forward vision technique, where your eyes are steps ahead of your feet, anticipating or "setting up" for upcoming obstacles on trail descents, helps you select a line in the trail that, in turn, helps you to maintain speed without losing balance or twisting an ankle.

Depending on running style, the length of the run, and the distance traveled, trail runners may find it easiest to use a shorter stride and to run through rough footing with lighter but more rapid steps. Running on your forefoot, the way football players—hardly known for their daintiness— run through tire obstacle courses, takes weight off your feet so you can quickly adjust your balance and recover from any misstep. Of course, this is difficult to do when tired and legs and feet feel heavy and sluggish.

Trail runners will probably always wonder whether it is best to jump over, go around, or step on top of a fallen tree, branch, rock, or other obstacle blocking the most direct line of travel along a trail. Even though the decision to jump is driven by numerous factors, trail runners must make the choice instantaneously. Some of the more substantial variables in the equation are the speed at which you approach the obstacle, the size and stability of the obstacle, your general agility and experience, the footing leading to and from the obstacle, and your general level of chutzpah or cunning.

Once you've made the lightning-fast decision of whether to go over or around an obstacle, embrace it with confidence, then leap over, step on, or steer around the barrier without second-guessing the decision. Don't dwell on a botched decision, but learn from mistakes so as to be better able to tackle the next trail barrier. The element of surprise, the challenge of uncertainty, and the never-ending supply of different obstacles are what make trail running exciting. If these uncertainties do not make for fun and excitement, run roads.

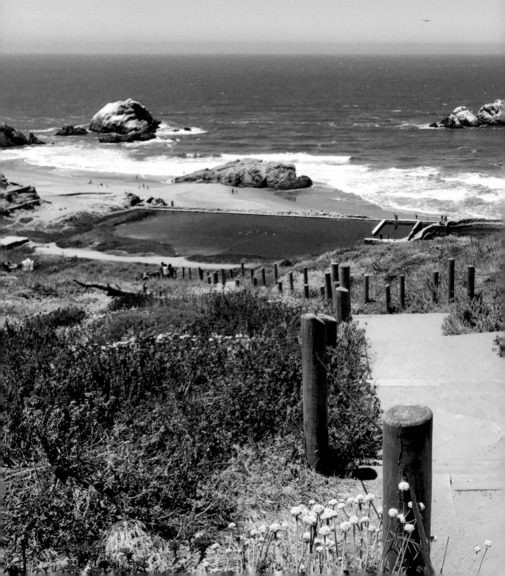

SAN FRANCISCO

LANDS END

ON THE NORTHWEST END OF SAN FRANCISCO, just east of the Cliff House, is Lands End, which is operated by the Golden Gate National Recreation Area. The trails are shaded by the many cypress trees, but do stay on the trails, as there are cliffs with 200-foot drops into the Pacific Ocean. The trails afford views of the Golden Gate Bridge and Marin. In spring the wildflowers are in bloom.

EL CAMINO DEL MAR TRAIL TO COASTAL TRAIL

THE RUNDOWN

START: Lands End parking lot; elevation 174 feet

OVERALL DISTANCE: 4.15 miles

APPROXIMATE RUNNING TIME: 50 minutes

DIFFICULTY: Lightly moderate

ELEVATION GAIN: 463 feet

BEST SEASON TO RUN: Year-round

DOG FRIENDLY: Yes. Dogs must be on leash or under voice control.

PARKING: Free

OTHER USERS: Bicyclists

CELL PHONE COVERAGE: Excellent

MORE INFORMATION: www .nps.gov/goga/planyourvisit/ landsend.htm

FINDING THE TRAILHEAD

Coming from the east, take Geary Boulevard, which turns into Point Lobos Avenue after 43rd Avenue. After passing 48th Avenue, take the first entrance to the right to the parking lot. Coming from the south, take the Great Highway. After passing the Cliff House and Louis Restaurant, turn left into the parking lot. **Note:** Due to the high number of car

EL CAMINO DEL MAR TRAIL TO COASTAL TRAIL

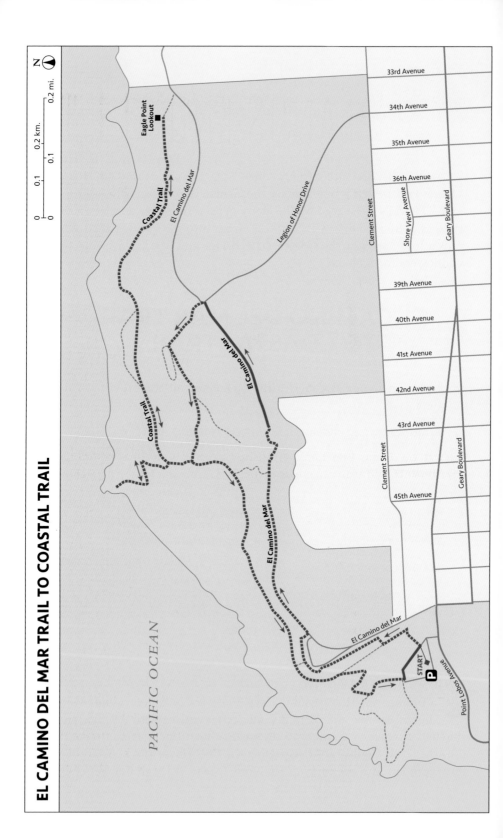

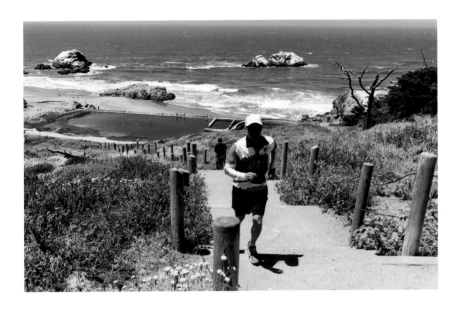

break-ins, carry your valuables with you and put all other items in your car trunk.

RUN DESCRIPTION

Start at the Lands End Lookout Visitor Center, which has restrooms, refreshments, and water. Go east through the parking lot until reaching a set of stairs. At the top of the stairs, continue east and turn left to run on the path adjacent to El Camino del Mar. Upon reaching the parking lot at a quarter of a mile, view the USS *San Francisco* Memorial and, just a few yards beyond, an overlook of the Golden Gate Bridge. The path to the southeast offers a view of the ropes course and West Fort Miley battery gun emplacements. Continue east on the sidewalk, which leads to a closed-off road. Follow the road for half a mile, where it turns into a trail, and continue for about a quarter mile to reach a set of stairs. Go up the stairs, leading to a road, and at the top of the hill, the 1-mile point, the route comes across the Legion of Honor Museum on the right. The path on the left is the paved Lands End Trail. Stay on the main paved trail through the golf course for a quarter mile and, at the bottom, turn right on the Coastal Trail, which used to be railroad tracks. Head east at 1.5 miles, ascending a set of rustic steps and then down the other side and up a small hill where the trail narrows. At Eagle's Point, at about 2 miles, turn around and head west on the same trail. Or you could continue onto El Camino del Mar to the Golden Gate Bridge. At 2.8 miles turn right and go down a somewhat steep and sandy path; near the bottom go left to check out the Mile Rock Beach or right to view the man-made rock formation dubbed the Labyrinth, and then retrace your steps to return to the top. At the top turn right and continue on the Coastal Trail. At 3.7 miles stay right and immediately turn right on a dirt path running straight to the finish or, after a few yards, turn right to go down the path to Sutro Baths. If the tide is low, it is possible to run south on the beach. Run past the baths and go up the stairs toward the parking lot. At the top turn right to end at the visitor center.

Along the coast, the Lands End, Coastal Trails, and Fort Funston Loop can be connected by running along Ocean Beach or the Great Highway (which can be driven as well).

COASTAL TRAIL WITH BATTERIES TO BLUFF OPTION IN THE PRESIDIO

JUST SOUTH OF THE GOLDEN BRIDGE, the Coastal Trail takes in views of the western portion of San Francisco and the Pacific Ocean. This route starts with some challenging footing on Baker Beach, followed by a hike up the infamous Sand Ladder. There is an option to run across the Golden Gate Bridge to add a few more miles, and an opportunity to explore the coastal fortifications if returning south on the route.

THE RUNDOWN

START: Battery Chamberlin; elevation 40 feet

OVERALL DISTANCE: 2.8 miles

APPROXIMATE RUNNING TIME: 32 minutes

DIFFICULTY: Moderate

ELEVATION GAIN: 505 feet

BEST SEASON TO RUN: Year-round

DOG FRIENDLY: Dogs must be on leash for all trails except the Batteries to Bluff Trail, where dogs are forbidden.

PARKING: Free in parking lots and adjoining roads but may be difficult to find on warm to hot sunny days

OTHER USERS: Bikers, walkers, and dog walkers. On warm days nudists may be sunbathing at Baker and Marshall's Beaches.

CELL PHONE COVERAGE: Excellent

MORE INFORMATION: www .presidio.gov/trails/california -coastal-trail

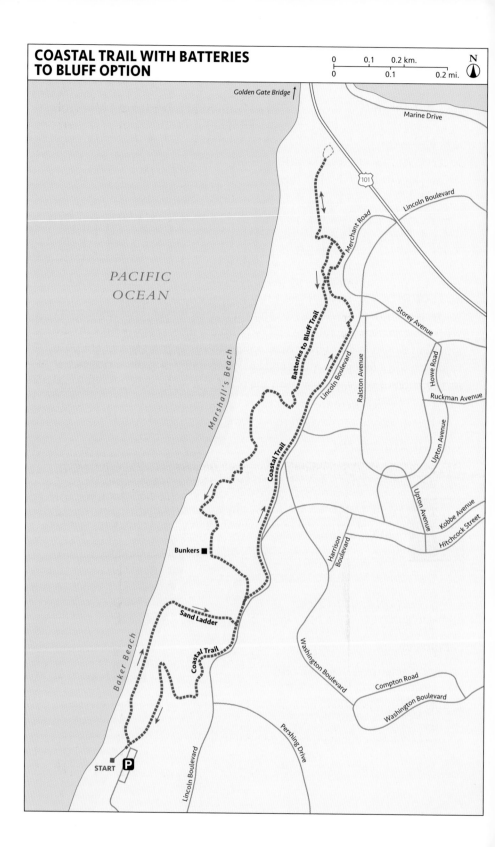

0   0.1   0.2 km.

0   0.1   0.2 mi.

N

Golden Gate Bridge

Marine Drive

101

Lincoln Boulevard

Merchant Road

PACIFIC
OCEAN

Storey Avenue

Howe Road

Ruckman Avenue

Batteries to Bluff Trail

Lincoln Boulevard

Ralston Avenue

Upton Avenue

Marshall's Beach

Coastal Trail

Upton Avenue

Kobbe Avenue

Hitchcock Street

Bunkers

Harrison Boulevard

Sand Ladder

Baker Beach

Coastal Trail

Washington Boulevard

Compton Road

Washington Boulevard

Pershing Drive

START P

Lincoln Boulevard

FINDING THE TRAILHEAD

Take 25th Avenue north. Turn right onto El Camino del Mar and enter the Presidio. The road turns into Lincoln Boulevard. Turn left onto Bowley Street. Enter Baker Beach. Just down the hill turn right onto Battery Chamberlin Road, which leads into a parking lot. Go north in the parking lot until you reach Battery Chamberlin.

RUN DESCRIPTION

Starting at Battery Chamberlin, go left and take the trail that leads to Baker Beach. Go north on the beach and run a half mile and turn right to go up the Sand Ladder, made infamous as part of the run course for the Escape from Alcatraz Triathlon. It's so steep, even the pros walk up this ladder, which comprises 200 10-foot poles tied together to form the stairs. At the top of the Sand Ladder, turn left and go up the Coastal Trail, which is adjacent to Lincoln Boulevard. Just past the Pacific Overlook, stay to the right (ignore the sign on the left trail indicating the way to Golden Gate Bridge). The trail curves left for a view of the Golden Gate Bridge and the parking lot. Cross over the bridge that goes over the bunkers and continue running north. At 1.3 miles there are two options: Continue underneath the Golden Gate Bridge and access the eastern walkway to run 2 miles and cross into

SAN FRANCISCO WEATHER

Many runners "let the weather be their coach," selecting their trail destination based on whether it is too wet and muddy or cold and icy. Forest runs are especially attractive as a cool respite from occasional hot and humid streaks. Occasional storms can bring strong rain and wind, and it is the latter that may make the forest a dangerous place. Having a tree fall on you can really ruin your day.

San Francisco runners know to carry adequate rainwear and to dress in layers, because the mistakes of the unprepared may result in uncomfortable—if not severe—lessons. Running with hydration may not be as obvious when there is abundant humidity, but for many of the longer routes we've included in this guide, you should bring fluids, especially if it is likely to take you longer than the projected time or if the day is a hot one.

Because of the likelihood of running across mud, your footwear selection can be crucial. Similarly, if you over- or underdress, that too may ruin your run. Be sure to get your layering dialed in from the outset.

Marin County, or continue east to access the waterfront. Otherwise, turn around. Just before crossing the bridge, take the stairs to the right that go over a battery. Run through the battery, heading down the stairs, and turn right to run through several more batteries. At 1.6 miles reach a fence and turn right to follow the Batteries to Bluff Trail. Go down the stairs to enjoy Marshall's Beach, then head back up a set of stairs to reach some bunkers. Run across the top of the bunkers to get to the trail that intersects the Coastal Trail. Turn left and go down past the entrance of the Sand Ladder. At 2.4 miles the trail turns away from Lincoln Boulevard and widens to a fire road. At the end of the fire road, just before the beach, make a hard left and go through the gate to run by Battery Chamberlin and finish the run. **Note:** If you don't want to run up the Sand Ladder, then just run the route in reverse.

FORT FUNSTON LOOP

LOCATED IN THE SOUTHWESTERN CORNER of San Francisco, Fort Funston was a former harbor defense installation and is now part of the Golden Gate National Recreation Area. Don't be surprised to see hang gliders in the skies overhead. Runs go by and through the fort's batteries, and the terrain includes sand dunes, making this short loop a little more challenging. However, the sandy annoyance is tempered greatly by views of the coastlines of San Francisco to the north and Pacifica to the south. Although the trails are not too well marked, it is hard to get lost due to the small area.

THE RUNDOWN

START: Fort Funston parking lot; elevation 180 feet

OVERALL DISTANCE: 2 miles

APPROXIMATE RUNNING TIME: 20 minutes

DIFFICULTY: Easy if you're used to running on sand

ELEVATION GAIN: 166 feet

BEST SEASON TO RUN: Year-round

DOG FRIENDLY: Yes, off-leash dogs allowed

PARKING: Free

OTHER USERS: Walkers

CELL PHONE COVERAGE: Excellent

MORE INFORMATION: www .nps.gov/goga/planyourvisit/ fortfunston.htm

FINDING THE TRAILHEAD

From I-280 take the John Daly Boulevard exit in Daly City. Turn and go west on John Daly until it dead-ends at Skyline Boulevard/ CA 35. Go right and head north for 1.5 miles. At the bottom of the hill where John Muir Drive meets Skyline, make a U-turn and go up the hill. At 0.4 mile the entrance to Fort Funston is on the right. Once in the park, turn right and park at the first visible building. The trailhead will be on the east, facing Lake Merced.

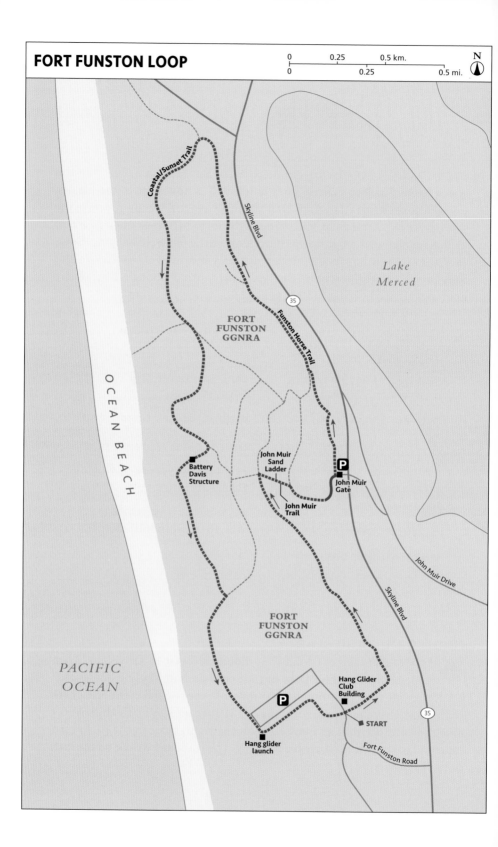

Coastal/Sunset Trail

Skyline Blvd

35

Lake Merced

FORT FUNSTON GGNRA

Funston Horse Trail

O C E A N   B E A C H

Battery Davis Structure

John Muir Sand Ladder

P

John Muir Gate

John Muir Trail

John Muir Drive

Skyline Blvd

FORT FUNSTON GGNRA

PACIFIC OCEAN

Hang Glider Club Building

P

START

35

Hang glider launch

Fort Funston Road

RUN DESCRIPTION

Starting on the Horse Trail located next to the Hang Glider Club building, go east very briefly and then turn left to go north on the sand. At the first intersection, veer right to follow the fence. After a third of a mile, turn right and head down a set of stairs, named the John Muir Sand Ladder. At the bottom of the stairs, turn right to run and downhill on the paved trail. At the bottom, you arrive at the John Muir Gate, where there are parking spaces. (**Note:** if you want to extend your run, cross the street and run the 4.5-mile paved loop around Lake Merced.) At this point take the unnamed sandy single track trail on the right, which is closest to Skyline Boulevard. Heading north, you will go slightly uphill and reconnect to the Horse Trail.

Just shy of 1 mile, you reach another fence and turn right to follow the fence in a counterclockwise direction. Upon reaching a paved path (if not covered with sand), turn left on the Coastal Trail (on some maps this trail is called the Sunset Trail) to go south. This trail alternates between pavement and sand dunes. (**Note:** Along the trail, there are a couple of entrances to Ocean Beach if you wish to run on the beach, but be sure to check the tide table to avoid running in times of high tide.) At 1.3 miles turn right and go uphill on the Coastal Trail/Sunset Trail. Upon reaching the Battery Davis structure, turn right (west) and go through its tunnel. Upon exiting the other end, turn left and follow the narrow, sandy path southward while enjoying soothing ocean sounds. Upon reaching the paved trail, turn right to continue south to finish at the parking lot, the spot from which hang gliders launch. Run along the parking lot back to where you started.

Note: Stay away from the cliffs, as dogs and humans have fallen off.

MOUNT SUTRO OPEN SPACE RESERVE/ INTERIOR GREENBELT TRAIL TOUR

THIS 80-ACRE AREA was developed by Adolf Sutro more than 100 years ago and sits just southeast of Golden Gate Park. The Mount Sutro Open Space is owned by the University of California, San Francisco, while the rest (Interior Greenbelt) on the northeast end is owned by the city of San Francisco. This area is home to towering eucalyptus trees with at least two dozen different bird species inhabiting them. The trails are singletrack and, like many in the Bay Area, are riddled with poison oak, which grows along the sides. The region gets considerable fog throughout the year, and the trail tends to be muddy. On those foggy days the run takes on an ethereal feel.

THE RUNDOWN

START: Johnstone Drive; elevation 705 feet

OVERALL DISTANCE: 3.1 miles

APPROXIMATE RUNNING TIME: 35 minutes

DIFFICULTY: Easy to moderate

ELEVATION GAIN: 741 feet

BEST SEASON TO RUN: Year-round (except during storms/ heavy rains due to the tall trees)

DOG FRIENDLY: Yes. Dogs must be on leash or under voice control.

PARKING: Free. Park along Clarendon Avenue. Do not park along Johnstone Drive or any of the adjoining streets, as the area is permit parking only. Be sure to secure your

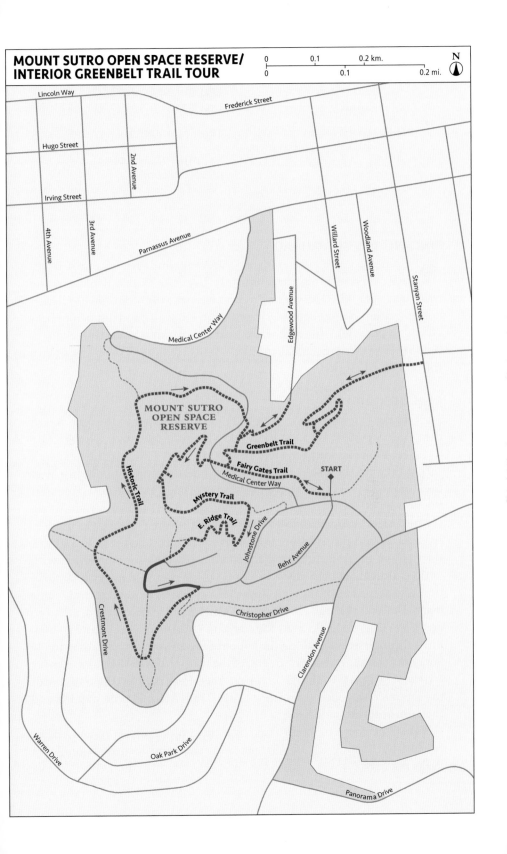

0   0.1   0.2 km.

0   0.1   0.2 mi.

N

Lincoln Way

Frederick Street

Hugo Street

2nd Avenue

Irving Street

4th Avenue

3rd Avenue

Parnassus Avenue

Willard Street

Woodland Avenue

Stanyan Street

Edgewood Avenue

Medical Center Way

MOUNT SUTRO
OPEN SPACE
RESERVE

Greenbelt Trail

Fairy Gates Trail

Medical Center Way

START

Historic Trail

Mystery Trail

E. Ridge Trail

Johnstone Drive

Behr Avenue

Crestmont Drive

Christopher Drive

Clarendon Avenue

Warren Drive

Oak Park Drive

Panorama Drive

valuables, as there have been car break-ins.

OTHER USERS: Mountain bikers, walkers, and dog walkers

CELL PHONE COVERAGE: Excellent

TRAIL MARKINGS: Very good

MORE INFORMATION: mntsutro.com

FINDING THE TRAILHEAD

From the north head south on 7th Avenue and turn left onto Clarendon Avenue. From the south take Lagunda Honda Boulevard and then turn right onto Clarendon Avenue. Near the top of the hill on Clarendon, take a left on Johnstone Drive. Within 100 yards, and just before Behr Avenue on the right, the trailhead is near the entrance to the University of California, San Francisco's Chancellor's residence. Sutro Tower is visible in the opposite direction.

RUN DESCRIPTION

Start on the Fairy Gates (or Topo) Trail and take a left at the fork. Reach the Upper Service Road and turn right to cross the road to the North Ridge Trail. At the next fork turn left on the Mystery Trail. At the next fork turn right onto the East Ridge Trail, which leads to the summit. Just after the summit stay left on the trail, heading through the Native Garden. At the bottom of the trail, enter the paved Nike Road and turn right down the hill. After running almost 1 mile, and just before reaching the residential area, turn right to follow the Quarry Trail. Just before mile 2 stay to the right on the trail and ascend for 0.1 mile, reaching an intersection with various trails. Take the Historic Trail, which goes in a northwest direction, and at the end of the trail cross the Upper Service Road at the 1.7-mile mark. Descend the trail to Woodland Canyon and make a hard left to go down the Edgewood Trail. At the end of the trail, turn around and go back up to the intersection, taking the left onto the Historic Trail leading to the Stanyan Street entrance. At the end of the trail, go down the stairs to enjoy a view of St. Ignatius Church in the distance. Head back up the trail, and at the intersection go left onto Fairy Gates Trail. After 0.1 mile stay left and then finish at the trailhead.

Note: The route to Twin Peaks is a third of a mile away and can be reached by turning left on Clarendon Avenue and then right on Twin Peaks Boulevard.

WHAT TO WEAR ON THE TRAIL

Trail runners often face the difficult "What am I going to wear?" dilemma when they look out the window before a run. With different layers of apparel, a trail runner can adjust during the run to moderate temperature, in response to both internal changes in exertion and external changes in weather. Technologically advanced fabrics have put a new twist to layering, elevating it to a modern art form, the object of which is to find the perfect balance of performance, temperature regulation, moisture control, insulation, and protection from exogenous elements such as wind, snow, and rain.

Layers can be broken into three primary categories: base (against the skin), mid (also known as the insulating, thermal, or performance layer), and outer (shell). While the following discussion is divided into these three categories, keep in mind that several manufacturers, mostly in the outdoor industry, have designed some excellent pieces of apparel that blur the layering distinctions by incorporating two or even all three layers into a single garment.

BASE LAYERS AND SOCKS

Worn next to your skin, base layers tend to be soft and are primarily designed to wick moisture from the skin while providing some warmth. Cotton, once very popular among runners as a base layer, is somewhat extinct as a performance fabric and is not recommended as a base layer because it retains moisture, does not breathe well, and becomes abrasive to skin when wet. In contrast, modern merino wool—which does not itch— is an ideal base layer material because it maintains dryness, helps regulate body temperature, and is resistant to bacteria.

The importance of an effective base layer must not be overlooked: A trail runner can wear the most advanced shell on the market, but it will be worthless if the runner is soaking wet on the inside.

Although a fabric's moisture management ability is important, the first priority in a base layer should be the material's ability to help regulate the body's microclimate. Ideally, a base layer maintains a sufficiently warm or cool temperature so that the runner is neither shivering nor sweating. By avoiding overheating, a runner will release less moisture, which helps to maintain better hydration and performance. Nonetheless, since perspiration is a natural component of exertion, an effective base layer regulates the body's microclimate by wicking moisture away from the skin so that it can evaporate or be passed through the mid and outer layers.

Base-layer fabrics wick moisture through one or a combination of chemical or mechanical techniques. Most technical synthetic base-layer fabrics are known as "hydrophobic," which means that they repel moisture instead of absorbing it. Polyester, nylon, and polypropylene are the most common hydrophobic fabrics used to draw moisture from the skin and repel it outward, where it evaporates if exposed to the air or transfers to a mid or outer layer, where it can be dispersed.

Base layers should be somewhat form-fitting or tight. Some moisture-wicking fabrics work best if they are snug against the skin. That contact allows them to wick moisture at an early stage. Some fabrics are even able to transport moisture while it is in the vapor state. Base layers should fit well with the trail runner's particular body type; and if chafing is a concern, select pieces that use flat seam construction.

When it comes to running in the cold, trail runners can keep their legs warm by choosing between tights and "loose tights" (also called "relaxed fit pants" or "track pants"), all of which are made from wicking base-layer fabrics with Lycra, Spandex, or other resilient materials blended in to make them soft, flexible, and quite warm. When it is really cold, double-layer tights, tights with windproof panels, or wind pants over tights usually keep the legs adequately warm. Whether wearing shorts, tights, or pants, consider wearing an underlayer of Lycra, Spandex, wind briefs, or wind shorts that feature strategically placed front microfiber panels to protect the more sensitive parts of the anatomy from chilling winds. Wearing fuller-cut undershorts as a base layer under tights or running shorts will also reduce inner-thigh chafe. Compression tights, due to their constriction of blood flow, may not have the desired thermal qualities of looser-fitting leggings.

Regardless of aesthetic preferences, the most important qualities in choosing socks for trail running are temperature regulation, moisture management, cushioning, and protection from blisters. Some trail runners prefer thin synthetic socks that have minimal cushioning and offer a better trail "feel." Others find that thicker wool socks maintain a comfortable foot temperature in varying weather, in wet conditions, or on trail runs with water crossings. Those concerned about cushioning may opt for socks that are constructed with various weave patterns in different zones of the footbed to enhance cushioning and comfort. Some trail runners use trail shoes that feature relatively firm midsoles, and temper that rigidity with cushioned socks.

MID LAYER

The second layer, known as the mid, thermal, or performance layer, is a continuation of the base layer in managing moisture. The mid layer also provides thermal insulation. Mid layers work with the base layer to transfer moisture to the outer layer and are often made of the same hydrophobic materials, but with a more spacious weave. Fleece, especially microfiber fleece, works well as a mid layer because it has moisture-transfer qualities, boasts a high warmth-to-weight ratio, and is not bulky. Some thermal-layer fabrics use quilted weaves or other patterns that incorporate air pockets for increased warmth.

OUTERWEAR

Finding an ideal outer layer or shell presents the problem of balancing and achieving both breathability and weather resistance. With the goal of keeping you warm and dry by resisting or blocking the elements, such as wind, rain, or snow, the shell must also allow perspiration to escape through vents and technical features of the fabric. Except under extreme conditions, totally waterproof fabrics are overkill and even undesirable for trail runners. Waterproof materials tend to add bulk, inflexibility, expense, and especially reduced breathability to the garment. A stormproof outer layer sounds great for trail runners who confront freezing rain, but if their jackets and pants do not breathe well, those runners quickly become as wet from the inside as they would have had they chosen shells that lacked any water-resistant properties.

In most conditions trail runners will be served best by wearing microfiber outer layers that allow molecules of body-temperature vapor to escape while being windproof and water resistant rather than waterproof. Microfiber garments are often less expensive, weigh less, pack smaller, and are more pliant and therefore less noisy than their waterproof counterparts. Some manufacturers have applied laminates or encapsulating processes to enhance the windproof qualities and water-resisting performance of microfiber apparel.

Important qualities that distinguish functional trail-running shells from those that are better used for other types of outdoor recreation include the presence and optimum placement of venting systems, pockets, hoods, cuffs, closures, lining, and abrasion-resistant panels. When considering the purchase of a jacket with all the bells and whistles, think about whether the weight and cost of each zippered, snapped, Velcroed, or cord-locked opening is necessary.

Decide what style of shell—pullover "shirts," full-zip jackets, or vests—is best. Also consider the costs and benefits of such features as self-storage pockets and the integration of other fabrics in various panels, such as fleece, stretch material, breathable material, wicking material, or mesh back sections. If night running in proximity to motor vehicles is part of the regime, reflective taping is a worthwhile feature. Finally, try on the jacket to check the collar height, and look for the presence of a fleece chin cover to protect from exposure to or abrasion from cold zipper pulls.

Head and Hands

Trail runners should think twice before setting out on a jaunt without a hat, cap, or neck gaiter. Caps, especially those with bills, protect the scalp and eyes from sun and reduce the chances of overheating. Many caps are made out of moisture-wicking materials, and some feature mesh sides for venting heat. Some hats are made specifically for blocking the sun, having been constructed of fabric with a high SPF rating, and feature draped flaps that shield the neck from sun rays. Neck gaiters are multifunctional. They can be worn loosely around the neck or worn on the wrist, as a scarf, to cover the ears, or can be fashioned like a balaclava.

Given that approximately half the body's heat escapes through the head, hats are the single most important item of apparel for maintaining warmth. Many hats can be rolled up or down to expose or cover ears as a means of adjusting for a more comfortable temperature. When running in extreme cold, look for hats that are made with fleece, wind-blocking materials, wool, or combinations of fabrics that preserve warmth yet wick away perspiration under a variety of foul weather conditions. When the temperature is particularly frigid or if the windchill factor makes exposure and frostbite a real danger, it may be necessary to run with a face covering, neck gaiter, or balaclava to protect skin.

Mittens are much warmer than gloves; and if manual dexterity is not a concern, mittens are probably a better choice for colder climes. Some trail runners wear bicycling or weightlifting gloves with padded palms to protect their hands from falls or when scrambling.

Gloves and mittens are made in a variety of different fabrics and vary in thickness. Some are made of moisture-wicking, windproof, or waterproof fabrics, while others feature high-tech materials that are either integrated into or coat glove or mitten linings to maintain a comfortable temperature. If the hand temperature rises above the engineered comfort zone or "target" temperature, the material absorbs the heat and stores it for subsequent release should the hands cool below the target temperature. As a final consideration, if the backs of mittens or gloves are likely to be used as a nose wipe, make sure the fabric is soft.

GOLDEN GATE PARK

OPERATED BY THE SAN FRANCISCO RECREATION AND PARKS, Golden Gate Park comprises 1,017 acres, making it larger than New York City's 843-acre Central Park. More than 13 million visitors come to the park each year to enjoy the gardens, cultural venues, lakes, and perhaps a ride on the carousel. Starting at the western end of the park where it meets the Pacific Ocean, this route utilizes most of the trails in the park and also crosses active roadways. Automobiles have the right-of-way, so be alert when coming out of the wooded areas and crossing the roads.

GOLDEN GATE PARK TRAILS

THE RUNDOWN

START: Beach Chalet parking lot; elevation 30 feet

OVERALL DISTANCE: 7.5 miles

APPROXIMATE RUNNING TIME: 90 minutes

DIFFICULTY: Easy

ELEVATION GAIN: 543 feet

BEST SEASON TO RUN: Year-round

DOG FRIENDLY: Yes. Dogs must be on leash or under voice control.

PARKING: Free. Park in the lots along Ocean Beach.

OTHER USERS: Bikers, Frisbee throwers, and walkers

CELL PHONE COVERAGE: Excellent

TRAIL MARKINGS: None. The trails are unnamed. However, the park is only a half mile wide, so it is nearly impossible to get lost, as the trails are bracketed by roads.

MORE INFORMATION: sfrecpark.org/parks-open -spaces/golden-gate-park -guide/

GOLDEN GATE PARK

N

1 mi.

1 km.

0.5

0.5

0.5

0

0

5th Avenue

5th Avenue

7th Avenue

9th Avenue

10th Avenue

Nancy Pelosi Drive

Bowling Green Drive

San Francisco Botanical Garden

Funston Avenue

15th Avenue

John F. Kennedy Drive

Lincoln Way

20th Avenue

Strawberry Hill

GOLDEN GATE PARK

Parnassus Avenue

23rd Avenue

Geary Boulevard

Balboa Street

Cabrillo Street

Fulton Street

John F. Kennedy Drive

Martin Luther King Jr. Drive

Irving Street

Kirkham Street

Lawton Street

30th Avenue

30th Avenue

35th Avenue

Sunset Boulevard

40th Avenue

Chain of Lakes Dr.

John F. Kennedy Drive

45th Avenue

La PLaya Street

START

P

FINDING THE TRAILHEAD

 Use the Beach Chalet parking lot off the Great Highway on the west side of the park, where there is water and a restroom.

RUN DESCRIPTION

Go north through the parking lot and cross John F. Kennedy (JFK) Drive to the Dutch King Day windmill. Facing north, take the trail to the right. After 0.1 mile turn right. The trail will parallel Fulton Street on the left. Just after crossing 47th Avenue, take the trail to the left. At the half-mile mark run on the roadway for 0.1 mile adjacent to the northern end of the Chain of Lakes. After crossing Chain of Lakes Drive East, continue back on the trail. At the three-quarter-mile mark at the west end of the dog training field, turn left and go southward down a short hill. Turn left and go east and follow the path that is adjacent to the bison paddock. At the 1-mile point exit the trail and cross 36th Avenue to be on the west end of Spreckles Lake. Follow the lake in a clockwise direction. At the northeastern end of the lake, go on the trail that is a part of a Frisbee golf course. Cross 25th Avenue and continue on the trail. At the 1.3-mile point at 25th Avenue, turn right and follow the path adjacent to Crossover Drive. At the 1.6-mile point there will be a water fountain on the right. Turn left and take the pathway adjacent to JFK Drive. Pass Rainbow Falls and immediately turn left at the sign for Prayer Book Cross. Within 20 yards take the path to the right. (The path to the left goes to the top of the hill to Prayer Book Crosshill.) The path will be adjacent to Park Presidio Bypass Drive. At the 2.5-mile point arrive at the Rose Garden. Continue east back on the trail and turn left just after the 10th Avenue pathway, heading east past the playground. Go through two tunnels and enter the Music Concourse, then continue south through a third tunnel. Take any of the paved pathways eastward through Rhododendron Dell and take the trail exiting briefly on JFK Drive to get a view of the Conservatory of Flowers, then turn right onto the trail. Go up a slight hill and follow the path east along Lily Pond. Cross over Nancy Pelosi Drive and turn right to go east.

At the 3.5-mile mark arrive at the AIDS Memorial Grove and go west through the grove. At the end of the grove, take the middle path and go up. At the top take the path to the right and then turn left to go west on Pelosi Drive at the 3.9-mile point. At the end of Pelosi Drive, turn right onto Martin Luther King (MLK) Drive, which will take you past the Shakespeare Garden followed by the Japanese Tea Garden. On the right there will be several paths that you can take to do a mile loop around Stow Lake or to go up Strawberry Hill. Cross 19th Avenue. Cross Traverse Drive and turn right at the water fountain. Follow Traverse Drive and take the first trail on your left, leading to Elk Glen Lake. Turn right at the lake and follow the lake counterclockwise. Take the path uphill to enter onto Middle Drive and turn left to go westward and downhill. At the west end of the Polo Fields, turn right and take the dirt path. Just as you are turning eastward, turn left on a trail going down and then turn right to run through Little Speedway Meadow. (**Note:** You will be running part of a national cross-country course in reverse.) Just before the parking lot, turn right to follow the sandy trail. Exit at the intersection of JFK Drive and Chain of Lakes Drive. Go west on JFK. At the end of the road, cross the street and enter the trail. Exit at MLK Drive. At the Murphy Windmill turn right, and the path will take you to the back side of the Beach Chalet. Enjoy a drink at their brewery.

STOW LAKE

THE RUNDOWN

START: Stow Lake Boathouse; elevation 290 feet

OVERALL DISTANCE: 2.2 miles

APPROXIMATE RUNNING TIME: 25 minutes

DIFFICULTY: Easy to moderate

ELEVATION GAIN: 148 feet

BEST SEASON TO RUN: Year-round

DOG FRIENDLY: Yes. Dogs must be under voice control.

PARKING: Free. Park along the lake or at the boathouse.

OTHER USERS: Bikers, walkers

CELL PHONE COVERAGE: Excellent

MORE INFORMATION: golden gatepark.com/strawberry-hill .html

FINDING THE TRAILHEAD

From the south take 19th Avenue north. Once in the park, turn right on Martin Luther King Drive. At the first available left turn, turn onto Stow Lake Drive. After 0.5 mile arrive at the boathouse. From the north enter the park at 8th Avenue and Fulton Street. At the stop sign turn right onto John F. Kennedy Drive. Turn left onto Stow Lake Drive and arrive at the boathouse in a quarter mile.

RUN DESCRIPTION

Starting at the boathouse, run east, or clockwise, around the lake. After 0.1 mile turn right and go over the bridge. After crossing the bridge, turn left and pass by Huntington Falls and the Golden Gate Pavilion, a temple-like structure that was a gift to San Francisco from Taipei. After nearly circumnavigating the island, you will arrive at a fork in the trail. Turn right and head uphill. After a quarter mile reach the top of the waterfall and the reservoir. Turn left and continue up a short, steep segment and enjoy the view. Run down the path to the west, which will curve back down to the top of the waterfall. Continue down the hill and, at the bottom, go east for 100 yards, crossing the bridge that you first crossed when starting the run.

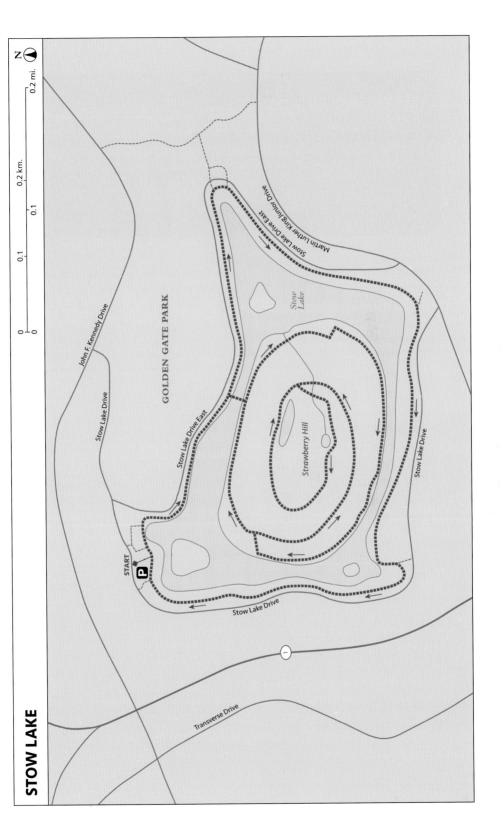

STOW LAKE

STRAWBERRY HILL

Rising nearly 430 feet, Strawberry Hill is a hill in the center of Golden Gate Park. The hill occupies an entire island in the park's man-made Stow Lake. The trail around the lake is paved. Boat rentals are an option following a run to enjoy the lake in a motorized or nonmotorized vessel. Although the trails are unmarked and unnamed, it is difficult to get lost because the trail is bracketed by the lake and the main road that goes around Stow Lake.

Once over the bridge, turn left to go back to the starting point, or turn right to run a clockwise flat mile back to the boathouse.

SIGN HILL PARK

SIGN HILL IS PART OF THE SAN BRUNO MOUNTAINS. When flying north from San Francisco International Airport or driving north on US 101, one can see the sign "South San Francisco the Industrial City" in white-painted concrete letters. The letters are set on the south side of a steep, 581-foot hill overlooking the city of South San Francisco. To create the appearance of straight, uniformly sized type despite the varied contour of the hillside, the letters are laid out anamorphically, ranging in height from 48 to 65 feet. The sign was created in the 1920s and is listed on the National Register of Historic Places. This run will take runners above, below, and up close to the letters. But there will be several steep sections for this short but unique route.

SIGN HILL PARK LOOP

THE RUNDOWN

START: Ridgeview Court parking lot; elevation 455 feet

OVERALL DISTANCE: 1.4-mile loop

APPROXIMATE RUNNING TIME: 20 minutes

DIFFICULTY: Moderate

ELEVATION GAIN: 596 feet

BEST SEASON TO RUN: Year-round

DOG FRIENDLY: Yes

PARKING: Free in parking lot or street parking

OTHER USERS: Mountain bikes on Ridge Trail only; walkers

CELL PHONE COVERAGE: Excellent

TRAIL MARKINGS: Good

MORE INFORMATION: www .ssf.net/departments/parks -recreation/parks-division/ sign-hill

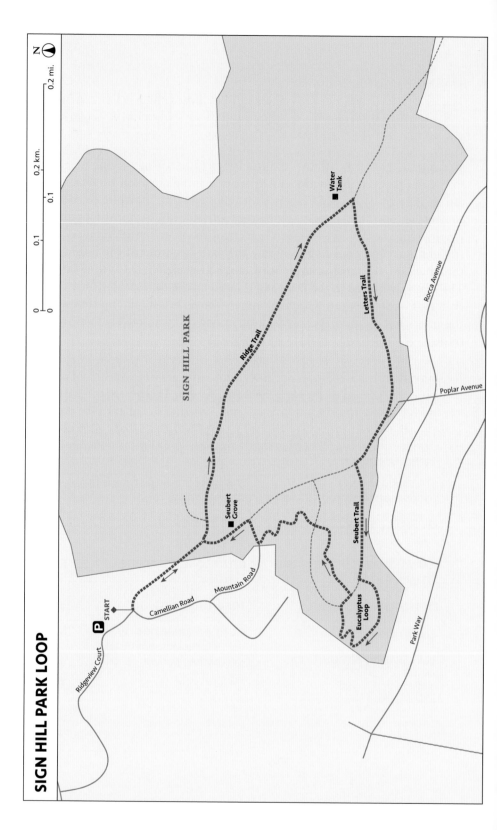

SIGN HILL PARK LOOP

FINDING THE TRAILHEAD

From I-280 get off at Westborough Boulevard and head east. After crossing El Camino Real, the street turns into Chestnut Avenue. At the fork in the road, turn right on Hillside Boulevard, then make a quick right onto Ridgeview Court and go uphill. The parking lot is across from the park entrance before the beginning of Carnelian Road.

RUN DESCRIPTION

Starting at the parking lot, enter the park and go up the paved path. After 0.1 mile, where the pavement ends, turn left and go upward and eastward on the Ridge Trail. You will hit the summit after a quarter mile of running. Enjoy the views and check out the sign below. Going down, you have a choice of taking the switchbacks or going straight and steeper. After a half mile turn right at Letters Trail, which is just before the water tank. At this point the trails are singletrack. On Letters Trail you can see the sign letters on your right and can veer off up the hill to check them out. After a half mile stay left to get to the Eucalyptus Loop. After the 0.1-mile loop, turn left and go uphill at the Eucalyptus Loop sign. For a third of a mile, the trail is steep and has stairs. At the top is Seubert Grove and the paved trail that you initially took to get to the Ridge Trail. Run down it or take the dirt path, which is about 20 yards to the right, to get back to the park entrance.

SAN FRANCISCO

APPENDIX A: ATRA RULES ON THE RUN

"Rules on the Run" are principles of trail-running etiquette that foster environmentally sound and socially responsible trail running. These principles emulate the well-established principles of Leave No Trace (https://lnt.org) and Rules of the Trail (www.imba.com/ride/imba-rules-of-the-trail) by the International Mountain Biking Association (IMBA). The American Trail Running Association (ATRA; www.trailrunner.com) believes that by educating trail runners to observe Rules on the Run, they will be able to enjoy continued access to their favorite trails and trail-running competitions.

1. **Stay on the Trail:** Well-marked trails already exist; they are not made on the day you head out for a run (i.e., making your own off-trail path). There is nothing cool about running off-trail, bushwhacking over and under trees, or cutting switchbacks up the side of a hill or mountain. Such running creates new trails, encourages others to follow in your footsteps (creating unmarked "social trails"), and increases the runner's footprint on the environment. When multiple trails exist, run on the one that is the most worn. Stay off closed trails, and obey all posted regulations.

2. **Run over Obstacles:** Run single file in the middle of a trail, even when muddy or laden with a fresh blanket of snow. Go through puddles and not around them. Running around mud, rocks, or downed tree limbs widens trails, impacts vegetation, and causes further and unnecessary erosion. Use caution when going over obstacles, but challenge yourself by staying in the middle of the trail. If the terrain is exceedingly muddy, refrain from running on the trails so that you don't create damaging "potholes" in the surface. Moisture is the chief factor that determines how traffic (from any user group) affects a trail. For some soil types a 100-pound runner can wreak havoc on a trail surface in extremely wet conditions. In dry conditions the same trail might easily withstand a 1,200-pound horse-rider combination. There are many situational factors to consider when making your trail-running decision. Trails that have been constructed with rock work or those with soils that drain quickly may hold up to wet conditions—even a downpour. But in general, if the trail is wet enough to become muddy and hold puddles, *all* user groups should avoid it until the moisture has drained.

3. **Run Only on Officially Designated Open Trails:** Respect trail and road closures and avoid trespassing on private land. Get permission first to enter and run on private land. Obtain permits or authorizations that may be required for some wilderness areas and managed trail systems. Leave gates as you've found them. If you open a gate, be sure to close it behind you. Make sure the trails you run on are officially designated routes, not user-created routes. When in doubt, ask the land managing agency or individuals responsible for the area you are using.

4. **Respect Animals:** Do not disturb or harass wildlife or livestock. Animals scared by your sudden approach may be dangerous. Give them plenty of room to adjust to you. Avoid trails that cross known wildlife havens during sensitive times such as nesting or mating. When passing horses, use special care and follow directions from the horseback riders. Running cattle is a serious offense. Consider turning around and going in another direction when faced with disturbing large herds of animals, especially in winter, when animals are highly stressed already.

5. **Keep Your Dog on a Leash:** Unless the area is otherwise posted, keep your dog on a leash and under control at all times. Dogs running off-leash may cause adverse impacts on terrain and wildlife and degrade the outdoor experience of other trail users. If an area is posted "No Dogs," obey signage. This may mean that you leave your dog at home. It is also imperative that you exercise Leave No Trace practices with respect to removing any dog waste, packing out what your dog may leave on the trail. Be prepared with a plastic bag, and carry the waste until you come across a proper disposal receptacle.

6. **Don't Startle Other Trail Users:** A quick-moving trail runner, especially one who seemingly emerges from out of nowhere on an unsuspecting trail user, can be quite alarming. Give a courteous and audible announcement well in advance of your presence and intention to pass hikers on the trail, stating something like "On your left" or "Trail" as you approach the trail users. Keep in mind that your announcement doesn't work well for those who are wearing headphones and blasting music. Show respect when passing others by slowing down or stopping if necessary to prevent accidental contact. Be ready to yield to all other trail users (bikers, hikers, horses) even if you have the posted right-of-way. Uphill runners yield to downhill runners in most situations.

7. **Be Friendly:** The next step after not startling fellow users is letting them know they have a friend on the trail. Friendly communication is the key when trail users are yielding to one another. A "Thank you" is fitting when others on the trail yield to you. A courteous "Hello, how are you?" shows kindness, which is particularly welcome.

8. **Don't Litter:** Pack out at least as much as you pack in. Gel wrappers with their little torn-off tops and old water bottles don't have a place on the trail. Consider wearing apparel with pockets that zip or a hydration pack that has a place to secure litter you find on the trail. Learn and use minimum-impact techniques to dispose of human waste.

9. **Run in Small Groups:** Split larger groups into smaller groups. Larger groups can be very intimidating to hikers and have a greater environmental impact on trails. Most trail systems, parks, and wilderness areas have limits on group size. Familiarize yourself with the controlling policy and honor it.

10. **Safety:** Know the area where you plan to run, and let at least one other person know where you are planning to run and when you expect to return. Run with a buddy if possible. Take a map with you in unfamiliar areas. Be prepared for the weather and conditions prevailing when you start your run, and plan for the worst, given the likely duration of your run. Carry plenty of water, electrolyte replacement drink, or snacks for longer runs. Rescue efforts can be treacherous in remote areas. ATRA does not advise the use of headphones or iPods. The wearer typically hears nothing around them, including approaching wildlife and other humans. The most important safety aspect is to know and respect your limits. Report unusually dangerous, unsafe, or damaging conditions and activities to the proper authorities.

11. **Leave What You Find:** Leave natural or historic objects as you find them. This includes wildflowers and native grasses. Removing or collecting trail markers is serious vandalism that puts others at risk.

12. **Give Back:** Volunteer, support, and encourage others to participate in trail maintenance days.

Trail Race Etiquette for the Race Director and Competitor

A few runners simply running on a trail normally have limited negative impacts. All the associated happenings of a trail race "event" add up and contribute to the total impact.

PREPARING FOR THE RACE AND SELECTING A COURSE

1. Involve the community. Make sure you secure all permits, permissions, and insurance. Cooperation from government officials (which may include parks departments, USDA Forest Service, etc.) is a must. Be mindful of potential trail conflicts with other users, which may include hikers, bikers, equestrians, or hunters. Let other public trail and area users know of your event in advance by using the media, postings at trailheads, etc., so that they have a chance to avoid the area during your race and are not surprised by the presence of runners on race day.

2. Select a race course that uses officially designated open public trails. Trail runners may want to test the course before and after the event. Using existing trails has another benefit: The trail bed should be well established, durable, and firm. If you are using private trails or going through areas that are normally off-limits, let runners know this in advance, and strongly discourage them from using the route except on race day. Encourage your race participants to familiarize themselves with the race route only as much as is minimally necessary. Many popular race trails get "loved to death" during training by runners.

3. If existing trails don't offer the mileage or distance you would like to have as part of your course or the type of elevation gains or losses you need, adjust your race distance to accommodate what already exists. ATRA suggests that you always use existing trails rather than creating social trails or detours.

4. Think about spectator, crew, and media movement around the course. This can often cause more damage than actual racing. Post signs to direct spectators to other course sections via established paths.

5. Limit the total number of participants allowed in your event in advance. Do not be greedy and blindly accept the number of entrants you might get. Work with land-managing agencies to set a number that you, your staff, and the surrounding environment, trails, and

facilities can safely accommodate with limited impact. Strive for quality of runner experience first and quantity of runners later only if increased numbers can be accepted comfortably.

6. Consider encouraging carpooling to your race by allocating preferential parking areas to vehicles with three or more runners, giving cash "gas money" incentives to those runners who carpool, etc.

7. Realize that most people visiting a natural area where your trail race will be held are visiting that area primarily to experience natural sights, sounds, and smells. Most trail race participants value these experiences also. Carefully consider how any "additions" to your event will impact and modify the natural experience for your race participants and others. Do you really need amplified music at the start, finish, and aid stations? Will everyone appreciate cheering spectators? Are banners and mileage markers necessary? Can one course official silently standing at an intersection pointing the way take the place of numerous flagging and ground markings?

8. Consider the timing of your event so as not to conflict with other trail and area users during already heavily used time periods. Scheduling your event in the off-season may avoid potential conflicts.

9. Plan and position your aid stations to minimize conflicts with other users and to avoid environmental impacts. Locate them in areas where access is easy and durable or previously disturbed surfaces already exist, and away from areas favored by other users (campgrounds, fishing spots, picnic areas, etc.).

10. Plan your start/finish area with care. Is there adequate parking? Will heavy concentrated use damage the vegetation or land? Do restrooms already exist or can they be brought in and removed easily? Is there a wide enough trail (or better yet a road) for the first part of the race to allow the field to spread out and runners to pass before they separate enough to allow safe use of a singletrack trail?

11. If trail or start/finish/aid area conditions cannot accommodate your race without environmental damage (due to mud, high water, downed trees, etc.), consider canceling, rescheduling, or having an alternative route in place for your event.

12. Encourage electronic registration. Post your event entry forms online instead of printing and distributing thousands, or at least print entry forms on recycled paper.

DURING THE RACE

1. Mark the course with ecofriendly markings. These markings may include flour or cake mix (devil's food is great for courses run on snow), colored construction marking tape, paper plates hung on trees with directional arrows, or flagging. Remove all markings immediately following the race, but be sure your markers are still in place at race time so runners do not go off course.

2. Provide a large course map at the start/registration area so runners can familiarize themselves with the trail.

3. Don't allow participants to run with their dogs on the course. This is a safety issue for other participants and for the dogs. Dogs also have been known to tow runners to an unfair advantage in a race.

4. Use the race as an opportunity to educate runners and spectators about responsible trail running. Include information about responsible training and volunteerism in each racer's entry packet. If you have a race announcer, provide him or her with a variety of short public messages that talk about responsible use of trails, joining a trail-running club, and volunteering to maintain trails.

5. Encourage local trail advocacy organizations to share their information with the public at your event. If the race includes a product expo, allow local advocacy groups to exhibit without charge.

6. Green the event. Provide adequate portable toilets, drinking water, and trash receptacles. Let runners know where these will be located in advance. Recycle all cans, bottles, paper, and glass. Consider recyclable materials for awards and organic T-shirts for participants. Event organizers and all participants will benefit if they are seen as being at the forefront of energy and materials conservation. As a participant, carry a water bottle and refill at the aid station so you are not using extra cups. As a race director, consider requiring participants to start the race with their own fluid and food in a container (water bottle or pack) so as to eliminate the need for cups along the trail. Pack out your gel wrappers and trash. You as the participant should be responsible for your trash.

7. Limit spectator and crew access to points along the course that can safely accommodate them and their vehicles without damage.

Consider prohibiting all spectator and crew access to the trail to preserve the trail experience for the participants and to limit impacts.

8. Promote local recreational trail running by making sure that maps, guidebooks, and brochures are available at the race. Involve local schoolchildren in the event in a kids' run if you have the resources.

9. Stop to help others in need, even while racing, and sacrifice your own event to aid other trail users who might be in trouble.

10. ATRA suggests that participants refrain from using iPods/headphones in races. This is foremost a safety issue. Many running insurance providers do not permit use of these devices.

11. When you have two-way traffic, slower runners yield to faster runners, and on ascent/descents the uphill runner should yield to the downhill runner.

12. Try to be patient when you are part of a conga line on crowded racing trails. Instead of creating social trails by passing a runner above or below the marked trail, yell out "Trail" and "To your left" or "To your right." If you are the slower runner, stop and step aside to make it easier for the faster runner to overtake you.

13. ATRA does not condone bandit runners (unregistered runners). Not only are bandits a serious safety and liability concern for the race director, often there are limits in races set forth by a permit. Bandits can jeopardize the issuance of future permits.

14. Require runners to follow all race rules, including staying on the designated marked route, packing out everything they started the race with, not having crew/pacers/spectators on the route, etc. Send a strong statement by disqualifying those runners who do not follow the rules.

AFTER THE RACE

1. Do a thorough job of cleaning the start/finish area and parking lots and repairing and restoring the trails used for the event. Leave the trails in better shape than they were prior to the race. Document your restoration work with photos.

2. If your event has been financially successful, make a contribution to your local trail-running advocacy group and, if possible, to ATRA,

too. When you do this, send press releases announcing your dona-
tions. This will enhance your image in the local community.

3. Get a capable runner to run sweep of your entire race route as soon
   as possible after the event. This runner can pick up trash and course
   markings, note any trail damage that needs to be mitigated, gauge
   reaction from other trail users they encounter, as well as act as a safety
   net. This runner should carry a pack, cell phone, first-aid kit, etc.

APPENDIX B: ROAD RUNNERS CLUB OF AMERICA GENERAL RUNNING SAFETY TIPS

- **Don't wear headphones.** Use your ears to be aware of your surroundings. Your ears may help you avoid dangers your eyes may miss during evening or early-morning runs.

- **Run against traffic so you can observe approaching automobiles.** By facing oncoming traffic, you may be able to react quicker than if it is behind you.

- **Look both ways before crossing.** Be sure the driver of a car acknowledges your right-of-way before crossing in front of a vehicle. Obey traffic signals.

- **Carry identification or write your name, phone number, and blood type on the inside sole of your running shoe.** Include any important medical information.

- **Always stay alert and aware of what's going on around you.** The more aware you are, the less vulnerable you are.

- **Carry a cell phone or change for a phone call.** Know the locations of public phones along your regular route.

- **Trust your intuition about a person or an area.** React on your intuition and avoid a person or situation if you're unsure. If something tells you a situation is not "right," it isn't.

- **Alter or vary your running route pattern; run in familiar areas if possible.** In unfamiliar areas, such as while traveling, contact a local chapter of Road Runners Club of America or a local running store. Know where open businesses or stores are located in case of emergency.

- **Run with a partner.** Run with a dog.

- **Write down or leave word of the direction of your run.** Tell friends and family of your favorite running routes.

- **Avoid unpopulated areas, deserted streets, and overgrown trails.** Avoid unlit areas, especially at night. Run clear of parked cars or bushes.

- **Ignore verbal harassment and do not verbally harass others.** Use discretion in acknowledging strangers. Look directly at others and be observant, but keep your distance and keep moving.

- **Wear reflective material if you must run before dawn or after dark.** Avoid running on the street when it is dark.

- **Practice memorizing license tags or identifying characteristics of strangers.**

For more information, go to www.rrca.org.

APPENDIX C: USEFUL WEBSITES

www.trailrunner.com

www.trailrunproject.com

www.strava.com

Bay Trail Runners: www.baytrailrunners.com/

Brazen Racing: https://brazenracing.com/

Coastal Trail Runs: www.coastaltrailruns.com/

Dirt Dog Trail Runners: www.dirtdogtrailrunners.com/

EnviroSports: www.envirosports.com

Inside Trail: http://insidetrail.com/

Pacific Coast Trail Runs: http://pctrailruns.com/

Sasquatch Racing: www.sasquatchracing.com/

Troy's California Trail Runs: www.tctruns.com/

Urban Coyote Racing: www.urbancoyoteracing.com/

Wolf Pack Events: http://wolfpackevents.com/calendar/142

BAUR (Bay Area Ultra Runners): www.run100s.com/BAUR/

Scena Performance series: http://scenaperformance.com/

Singletrack Running series (e.g., Folsom Lake Ultra): http://singletrack running.com

NorCalUltras: www.norcalultras.com/

Ragnar Relay series: www.runragnar.com/